SELF-ESTEEM

WORKBOOK

*A Practical Guide to Help You
Overcome Self-Doubt and
Insecurity, Gain Better
Confidence and Inner Strength.
Discover Your Hidden Potential
and Change Your Life in 30
Days*

Dalton McKay

Table of Contents

Introduction

Welcome to *Self-Esteem Workbook: A Practical Guide to Help You Overcome Self-Doubt and Insecurity, Gain Better Confidence and Inner Strength — Discover Your Hidden Potential and Change Your Life in 30 Days.* Thank you for choosing this book. It was written with the intention of helping you improve your self-esteem and personal skills.

There may be times that you feel like life is difficult, especially when things aren't going your way. It is perfectly normal to go through ups and downs in life. The fact of the matter is that success does not come without obstacles. Rather, success comes from the life that you lead in spite of the issues and problems that you might have.

This book has been written with the average person in mind. You will find strategies that can help you to overcome unpleasant roadblocks in your life. For instance, you might have a habit or two that you would like to get rid of. It is certainly worthwhile to look at how you can replace a negative habit with a more positive one.

At the end of the day, this is what life is all about: achieving your goals and dreams. Whatever they are, your dreams are the most important thing that you can focus on in life. Now, this doesn't mean that you are going to be acting selfishly. Your goals, as ambitious as they might be, may be centered on your family, your community, and of course, yourself. That is certainly something to strive for and fight for each and every day.

In this book, you will find practical strategies that can help you overcome any of the roadblocks that might be standing in your way. Perhaps you've tried to do this before. Perhaps you have been unsuccessful in those past attempts. This book promises you can succeed at practically anything in as little as 30 days.

Yes, that's right, 30 days.

There is no magic and no gimmicks. Everything you will find in the book is based on solid logic, common-sense experience, and science. If you have encountered experts and gurus who make outrageous claims about turning people's lives around at the drop of a hat, then you know how important it is to have a sound approach that is sustainable in the long-term.

Overall, we are going to be talking about how low self-esteem and low self-confidence. This information will help you pinpoint aspects in your life that may need to change. Additionally, we will go over ways in which you can address any personal weaknesses which you have identified. The practical strategies featured in this book are focused on contributing to your personal development.

Once you have taken on the strategies that we have developed, you will be able to translate them into a winning formula that can hold up over time. The best part about this is that you don't need any superpowers to achieve these goals. You already have everything it takes to become the successful person you have always wanted to be.

Perhaps the most important thing to keep in mind is that you need to act! You can't expect to see any progress without first making up your mind to change.

So, let's get started!

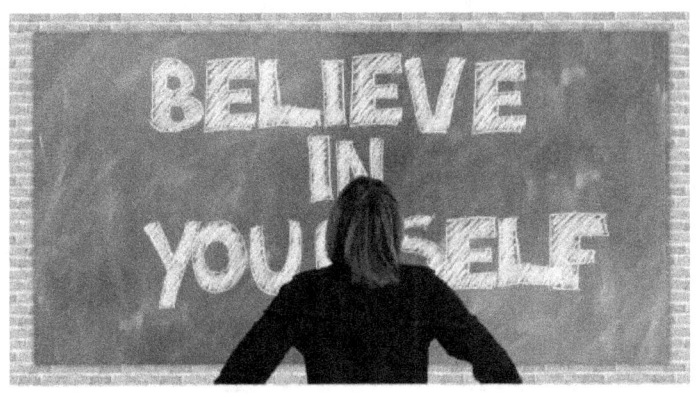

Part 1: What Is Self-Esteem and Why Is It Important?

Let's start this part with an explanation. This first part is quite theoretical and serves to provide a historical overview of studies done in the last century on this subject. Though this may not interest you, understanding the origin of the strategies you'll be using may help you to have the proper mindset. You can, of course, move on to the second chapter and maybe go back to reading this one later.

1. Abraham Maslow and the Theory of Human Motivation

Abraham Maslow is one of the most persuasive therapists of the twentieth century. His most recognized research was on the Hierarchy of Needs. Maslow's work in brain research began even before fundamental breakthroughs in brain research had developed. If it were not for him, everything would be much different.

The serious challenge in the present work sector puts the coherence of organizations in danger. Organizations require more execution and profitability to keep progressing, and this causes a burden on the representatives of the organizations. In present-day organizations, humans are a functioning labor force that can be affected by numerous components. Therefore, if performance and efficiency are required inside an organization, the labor force needs to be remotely motivated. External motivation is the motivation that speaks to the mission of an organization.

Motivation is an idea that has been known for centuries but has only started to be examined recently. Motivation is most important because of the benefits it gives. Therefore, it is critical for directors, educators, firm pioneers, mentors, social insurance providers, and guardians to put individuals into action. Individuals can be persuaded either because they respect a movement or as a result of strong external elements. Therefore, specialists that had come to understand the significance of the times when individuals were viewed as robots have further studied motivation and, as a result, created a different hypothesis.

The hypothesis of motivation was advanced by Maslow in the year 1943, and with this hypothesis, a hierarchy of requirements that influenced motivation was built up. Be that as it may, Abraham Maslow's theory of the order of human necessities appears at the front line of the most significant studies on motivation. No motivation hypothesis for the past several decades was taken to be as effective as Maslow's Hierarchy of Needs. The hypothesis set by Maslow argues that people are inspired not by external thought processes—for example, reward and discipline—but by internal needs. At the end of the day, needs come before the motivation that a person has.

Motivation is an idea that includes wants, drives, wishes, interests, and needs. Drive is motivation that is physiological—for example, thirst, hunger, or sexuality. Needs are great drives that are to be accomplished but are human-specific (Cüceloğlu, 2016). Maslow's hypothesis argues that the needs of humans are boundless—meaning that when one need is satisfied, another new need emerges. Every need is identified with fulfillment or disappointment of different needs, and unsatisfied needs are an incredible source of motivation for people.

The study is significant because it gives data and direction to leaders of different organizations to improve the motivation of their subordinates, which is one of the most fundamental strategies applied to boost performance and profitability in organizations. It carries a different point of view to the hypothetical questions and looks at the adjustments in Maslow's hypothesis.

Individuals have mental, biological and social perspectives and accordingly have specific and various needs. Those needs are able to fluctuate from person to person to pursue a leveled order that progresses from fundamental physiological needs towards mental and social needs. Maslow's Hierarchy of Needs, which is at the front line of the most significant investigations about motivation, has additionally made the "Pyramid of Hierarchy of Needs" by placing the requirements in a specific order, as illustrated in the figure below:

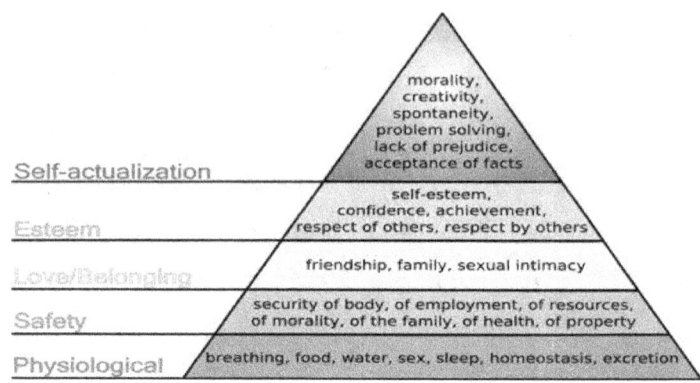

Physiological Needs: These are needs that must be satisfied in order for an individual's natural body structure to continue functioning—for example, shelter, sleeping, eating, taking water, and breathing in oxygen. Maslow depicted those necessities as physiological drives, and they started the motivation hypothesis and highlighted the need for it to include two essential focuses.

Human beings should first be supplied with water, minerals, salt, nutrients, sugar, fats, and proteins, etc. for homeostasis to take place. In any case, it is preposterous to define all the physiological needs with homeostasis. Some needs—such as taste, rest, smell, sex, and strength—are physiological needs, and not homeostatic. Needs that are physiological are usually obligatory.

On the off chance that they are not met, different needs won't jump out at an incredible degree. It can barely be argued that opportunity and popular government, workmanship, artistry, sports, and good quality music stand out, and they ought to in individuals and social orders that may not have fulfilled their mandatory needs (Maslow, 1954).

Safety Needs: Although the physiological needs are moderately satisfied, needs that are new come up and are classified as security needs (Maslow, 1943). Those are the necessities. For instance, having confidence, threat insurance, and lack of bad feelings. Being secure financially is another component of someone's wellbeing. The protection idea comes from a framework advantage. For instance, fire and food are some factors that depend on this need. The military and police associations of the networks are also because of their safety needs (Telimen, 1977; Eren, 2012). Furthermore, the safety needs can likewise advance as indicated by the social concerns or the states of the nation they live in.

Love and Belongingness Needs: When the physiological needs and security needs are completely met, the requirement for adoration, responsibility, and belongingness develops. People are social creatures (Stephens, 2000; Adair, 2013). People need to feel belongingness and love, and this need can be met in many areas of life. For example, sentiments of having a place such as clubs, houses of worship, business affiliations, and so on, or having a life partner or a child (Seeley, 1988). People need other people.

Esteem Needs: There are two sorts of esteem needs. The first is the need to be valued and regarded by others identified with the notoriety of an individual; for example, status, acknowledgment, and appreciation. The other one is simply the need for thankfulness and confidence; for example, self-confidence, freedom, achievement, and ability (Maslow, 1954, 2013).

Self-Actualization Needs: Even though every one of the requirements at different degrees of the progression is satisfied, the individual will feel uneasy and dissatisfied. Individuals ought to act as per their own capacities. An artist ought to participate in music, a craftsman ought to take part in workmanship, and a writer must write to be upbeat. An individual ought to be whatever the individual can be (Maslow, 1943). Self-acknowledgment is an effort made by a person to boost his or her own abilities, to build up his or her aptitudes, and to arrive at the perfect kind of individual he or she truly needs to be. Since this is a requirement for development, there is no immersion point, and the necessities increase in relation to their paces of fulfillment.

Maslow (1943; 1954) portrays individuals who acknowledge themselves as people with elevated levels of impression of the real world, ready to go about, tending to be separated from everyone else in light of acting naturally sufficient, autonomous, and ready to know about and welcome the delights of life. As indicated by Maslow (1943; 1954), satisfied necessities lose their significance as motivational components. Nonetheless, it is beyond the realm of imagination to expect to isolate the requirements with careful limits.

It need not bother with 100% fulfillment to have the option to move from a specific need to a higher one (Hodgetts, 2006). Individuals who are satisfied with some upper-level needs may sometimes feel lower-level needs. Particularly in crises such as war, infection, or cataclysmic events, lower-level needs might be at the front line as the person's primary focus is survival during these times. As per Maslow, while the extents are not sure, it is sufficient to fulfill 85%

of the physiological needs, 70% of the security needs, half of the affection and belongingness needs, 40% of the thankfulness and regard needs, and 10% of the self-realization needs (Maslow, 1954).

Maslow's order of necessities hypothesis has been canvassed by various examinations until today. McGregor's theory of X and Y and the hypothesis of Z made by Quichi were made with the effect of Maslow's Hierarchy of Needs. Theory X and Theory Y are two direct inverse speculations, and they clarify the practices administrators have been created by their recognitions about representatives. Z hypothesis contends that chiefs ought to precisely decide the frames of mind of representatives as per target criteria. The most significant accentuation in the hypothesis is that necessities may change, as indicated by time and circumstance (Quichi, 1982; McGregor, 2017).

While there have been countless studies proving Maslow's Hierarchy of Needs to be significant, it has been scrutinized, as well. Hanley and Abell (2002) have expressed that Maslow's progressive system of necessities tends toward the Western idea and that the hypothesis was condemned by the women's activist masterminds, existential thinkers, nature lovers, and others.

They likewise scrutinize that the hypothesis is completely self-awareness arranged. As per the creators, even though Maslow's hypothesis doesn't completely overlook the connections, it is inadequate seeing someone because uniqueness is given specific significance. Maslow, doing his investigations in the United States in a moderate, utilitarian condition commanded by upsetting work and fight, couldn't segregate himself from this social condition.

For instance, in an examination led in China, it was found that people fulfill their belongingness needs before everything, and in an investigation led in Turkey, the requirement for wellbeing precedes the physiological needs (Varoğlu et al., 2000; Yang, 2003). Frei (2004) contends that Maslow's hypothesis neglected to clarify the presence of feelings.

As per the hypothesis, feelings will most likely not exist until the lower-level needs like wellbeing are fulfilled. Eckerman (1968) contends that the requirement for "consistency," which has not been tended to in the hypothesis, shows itself as a significant hindrance in changing a person's conduct and ought to be included as the last advance in the hierarchy.

Ultimately, there are numerous professionals claiming that this need-based hypothesis is insufficient as far as clarifying the practices in working life. In an examination directed by Wofford (1971) in the USA, it was discovered that an elevated level of motivation was a progressively effective spark for workers who were not able to fulfill their low-level needs.

2. How Does Low Self-Esteem Develop?

In some research studies, confidence is seen as a continuum that can be said to be low, medium, or high—and it is frequently evaluated as a numerical digit. Both the low levels and the high levels have an ability to be socially and sincerely destructive to an individual when viewing them. It's definitely thought that the best degree of confidence lies in the continuum. Individuals that work in this kind of range are said to be somewhat more overwhelmed socially with connections inside.

We learn things in various manners. We may learn from direct encounters, the media, observing other individuals, and tuning into what individuals talk about. This will proceed for the duration of our lives, be that as it may, convictions about ourselves are frequently formed overtime starting from early childhood experiences. Important encounters in our youth from the community we lived in, the schools we went to, and the friends we played with, have impacted our considerations and convictions about a wide range of things, including ourselves.

If we have adopted exceptionally negative convictions about ourselves, almost certainly, we have experienced an assortment of negative encounters that contributed to this. Below are examples of possible negative encounters.

Abuse or Neglect: How we were treated by important people in our life influences the manner in which we see ourselves, otherwise known as our identity. If we were treated poorly, such as in the instance of being abused or neglected by a caregiver or partner, we are often left with mental scars that cause us to think less highly of ourselves (i.e. "I am damaged goods").

Trouble in Meeting Parents' Standards: Encountering harsh and consistent discipline or being held to unrealistically high standards can likewise have a negative impact. Some guardians and relatives are regularly centered around your shortcomings and rarely acknowledged your positive characteristics or triumphs (maybe making statements, for example, "You could have done better," or "That is bad enough"), making it difficult for you to acknowledge them yourself. Some guardians and relatives as often as possible prodded you, ridiculed you, and put you down, which could also contribute to a negative self-image.

Being Forced to Bear Other Individuals' Pressure or Trouble: Sometimes, when families experience unpleasant or upsetting life occasions, guardians may need to take an important role in managing the issues that have happened. Caregivers will most likely be unable to give a lot of consideration to their youngsters or kids as they are too overwhelmed. It is likewise conceivable that caregivers in such conditions become baffled, irate, on edge, or discouraged, and react accordingly to their youngsters, unfairly inviting them to share your distress.

Not Fitting in at Home or at School: A few people may have encountered the experience of being the 'oddball' at home or at school. They may have been less shrewd than their family or had various interests, gifts, or aptitudes different from others in the family (for example, being aesthetic, melodic, lively, or love arithmetic, science, expressions). Although they probably weren't scrutinized for their various advantages or capacities, these probably weren't recognized, appreciated, or accepted. At the same time, the accomplishments of their family or friends may have been admired or celebrated.

In that capacity, they may come to accept beliefs such as, "I seem to be strange," "I might be odd" or "I am mediocre."

An Absence of Positives: A lack of positive encounters in our lives can likewise influence our confidence. It may be that you didn't get enough consideration, acclaim, consolation, warmth, or fondness from loved ones. It may be the case that your essential needs were sufficiently met, but no more than that was given. A few guardians may have been sincerely far off, not physically tender, investing a ton of energy working (maybe to address the issues of the family) or on the other hand seeking after their own advantages and had almost no time with their kids. These encounters may impact how individuals see themselves, particularly in the event that they compare their encounters to their companions' who might have had more positive encounters.

3. How Does Low Self-Esteem Affect Us?

If you have low self-confidence because of entertaining negative thoughts about yourself, you will normally experience the following as a result:

- **More pressure and nervousness**- At the point in life in which one unable to visualize any amount of positive incentive in themselves and their capabilities, it's usually difficult for one to believe that they can deal with various demands in everyday life. Feeling that you will not and cannot satisfy such demands normally brings about a lot of pressure and tension.

- **A less beneficial and significant life**– By nature, the less worth that you identify in yourself and your life, the less your life feels beneficial, important, and worth living. Thus, low self-confidence can prompt melancholy and self-destructive coping mechanisms.

- **Pointless propensities** - In the event that you see practically no positive qualities in yourself, you will most likely not take care of yourself as well. This will also make you more likely to simply endure individuals mistreating you and not bother to fight back. On the off chance that you see loads of negative qualities in yourself, it may even lead you to loathe yourself, which at that point drives you to adopt approaches that ultimately hurt you even more.

- **Less satisfaction and delight throughout everyday life** - At the point when you see next to zero positive qualities in yourself, you are obviously no longer finding joy in things you once found joy in. You are unable to feel content or satisfied regardless of what you accomplished that day.

- **Less accomplishments in everyday life** - The less certain you are in your ability to do things thoroughly and correctly, the less likely you are to even attempt to accomplish what you need to accomplish in your day-to-day life. Basic tasks such as fetching a meal or getting dressed can feel impossible to do. Ultimately, this contributes to feeling poorly about ourselves.

- **Less fulfilling social interactions**– Those who do not think very highly of themselves are more likely to engage in social interactions that are unfulfilling and unproductive. This can be due to a lack of interest in meaningful, positive social interactions or a tendency to sabotage social interactions.

4. Short-Term Effects

Having a confidence level that is low may bring about damaging results, including but not limited to:

- High levels of stress and feeling anxious most of the time.

- Loneliness.

- Higher risk for depression resulting in issues with relationships including an inability to feel true connections, thus hindering us personally, socially, and professionally.

Besides all that, those antagonistic results can strengthen the contrary, mental way in which one does view themselves and brings an individual's self-confidence to an even lower level than it was.

5. Long-Term Effects

You Detest Your Body: A low level of confidence normally produces a poor body image. A poor body image can be powerful and has the potential to determine everything from how one reacts when they see someone to how one carries themselves at work. This can even prevent someone from prioritizing their wellbeing, as they probably feel they are unworthy of self-care.

You Loathe Yourself: There are moments in life when people feel disappointed and this is normal, but feeling that one hates themselves is a great indicator of a low level of confidence. Hating yourself is usually expressed by certain feelings of anger and dissatisfaction about one's identity and even a form of powerlessness to excuse oneself for even the slightest mistakes.

You're Fixated on Being Perfect: A more ruinous effect of a low level of confidence is perfectionism. A perfectionist is a person that lives with a constant feeling of being disappointed; despite having numerous accomplishments, they never feel good enough.

You're Oversensitive: One of the most difficult parts of a low level of confidence is being too sensitive. It can be troubling and lead to unnecessary conflict, resulting in even lower levels of self-confidence.

You Think You Don't Bring Anything to the Table: When we are uncertain of ourselves and start believing that we are useless perhaps as a result of harsh comments from others, we often do not participate in much because we believe we do not have anything to offer. This often results in us missing out on potentially meaningful interactions and experiences.

You're Frightful and on Edge: Feeling of dread and a conviction that you are weak against everything are undeniably connected to low self-confidence.

You Frequently Feel Furious: Anger and outrage are common and normal reactions, but happen more often and more intensely in the life of the person who is characterized by low self-confidence. When an individual starts to make unwise choices for themselves, then the individual begins to take in other people's sentiments and comments about them. Anger and hurtful feelings can develop when something very minor is experienced and causes outrage in an individual.

You're an Accommodating Person: Perhaps the most concerning issue with low self-confidence is feeling you need to satisfy others so that they like, love, and regard you. As a result, numerous accommodating people wind up feeling oppressed and used.

6. Benefits of a Healthy Self-Esteem

Analysis Loosens Its Hold: Analysis is valuable in certain instances, and someone with a healthy self-esteem can recognize that. Those without a healthy self-esteem often perceive analysis as criticism and grabs hold of anything to confirm their negative beliefs about themselves. It can turn life partners against one another, divide families, and sever important connections.

Mishaps Don't Get You Down: Indeed, even with a healthy self-esteem, you won't be resistant to the majority of life's inevitable mishaps. Actually, even with all the trust on the planet, you will likely still experience misfortunes, frustrations, and disappointments. The distinction? You may get knocked down, but you will have the solidarity to get back up and continue onward.

With low self-confidence, even the most minor stressor can feel like an enormous blow. In the context of relationships, this often leads to fights. Confronting each circumstance with confidence guarantees that regardless of what hand you're dealt, you will fearlessly face it. This also gives you that additional certainty to help you jump courageously into those enormous, new, and indeed, sometimes startling, experiences.

One of the hallmarks of having a healthy self-esteem is that adversity doesn't keep you down. When you are faced with a difficult situation, you are able to bounce back and come back stronger. The old saying, "it doesn't matter how many times you fall, but it matters how many times you get up" rings absolutely true. When your confidence is high, you can feel comfortable with negative circumstances. If anything, these uncomfortable experiences will provide you with a learning opportunity that you can't attain when things are easy.

You Can Express Yourself More Clearly: Is there anything in your life you'd like to attempt if disappointment wasn't a fear? Is it true that you are itching to say something but aren't sure how? Perhaps there's a fractured relationship you'd like to fix, yet you aren't certain you should attempt once more. Perhaps you're thinking about a lifelong change, yet don't think you have the means to return to school or to rejoin the workforce. That stone hindering you? It's your lack of self-confidence.

High self-confidence causes you to go after the things you need, request what you need, and express your real thoughts with more certainty. Studies demonstrate that numerous individuals, particularly ladies in the workforce, are reluctant to consult for a superior circumstance. Why? Individuals frequently tend to concentrate on the needs of others over their own. Building high self-confidence encourages you to focus on your own needs, giving yourself the spark you need to make that first move.

Your Relationships Are Healthier: With high self-confidence, you treat yourself better. You're additionally better equipped to maintain connections you need in your life. At the point when you're officially mindful of what you do and don't need - and better suited to verbalize those needs - you invite the positive energy you radiate. You are also more aware of those connections that are harmful and are more likely to sever them for your own good.

There's an immediate connection between domestic violence (in the entirety of its structures) and low self-confidence. Leaving isn't generally as straightforward as cutting off ties, so individuals who lack self-confidence also end up staying in abusive relationships. On the off chance that you or somebody you know is in an abusive relationship, the National Domestic Violence Hotline offers an accommodating Safety Plan to help you leave your abusive partner.

Overall, your self-confidence ends up playing a role in every facet of your important relationships. In the case of romantic relationships, you will find that your confidence will help you establish a healthy dynamic with your partner. A healthy dynamic may not have been a characteristic of your past relationships. But the fact of the matter is that your self-confidence and self-esteem will be able to garner the same amount of respect that you give. Since you won't be willing to let others take advantage of you, others will come to acknowledge that you are a worthy individual.

Still, the most important aspect of a healthy relationship, which is predicated by self-confidence, is the establishment of healthy boundaries. When you set healthy boundaries, you are able to not only give what you want, but also get what you want. This builds trust and respect, not to mention love and admiration. So, do make an effort to set healthy boundaries that can allow you to foster trust and understanding.

Stress Becomes More Manageable: As indicated by an ongoing review, most adults are worried about the burdens in their lives. From separation to family commitments to work obligations and everything in-between, it is easy to feel overwhelmed by all we need to manage. When we believe in our ability to handle what life throws at us, overwhelming stress becomes more manageable.

Then again, high self-confidence causes us to assemble the energy and assurance to face even the most unpleasant circumstance head-on. We're ready to fight off anything that causes us stress. From migraines and hypertension to anxiety and melancholy, stress can have serious effects on our bodies, wearing them out to the point of depletion. Moving toward upsetting circumstances with fearlessness and tirelessness can transform even the steepest mountain into a molehill.

Indeed, your mind can play tricks on you. When you have low self-confidence, your mind can get the best of you. You may begin to second-guess yourself or doubt your abilities. In fact, self-doubt can have such a stronghold on you that you may doubt your abilities, even when you have been successful in the past. This is why a high level of confidence can keep you grounded and feeling prepared, even when circumstances can lead you to doubt your own talents.

One other important point about having a high degree of confidence and self-esteem is that when things are looking tough, when the pressure is on, your belief in yourself will give you the edge you need when trying to manage.

That is one of the biggest advantages of relying on your own abilities.

Bliss: Teachers in learning institutions have observed that people that are fearless are always happier and more joyful with their lives compared to those who need constant validation and reassurance. Being confident in yourself can assist you in facing the world with more courage and energy, thus adopting and maintaining healthy and beneficial connections, doing work of good quality, as well as having a sense of belonging in the environment around you.

People that have healthy self-esteem are more effective in impacting other people's lives by just having the ability to have their feelings under control in order to tune into the feelings of others. In order to have an uplifting frame of mind, you should realize that you have an important role in the lives of others, and you matter.

Wellbeing: As per the Center of National Mental Health information, having high self-confidence and being certain are the factors that contribute to a better psychological state. A decent self-confidence is usually built when one is still young, and one's caregivers have some of the most long-lasting effects on their self-confidence.

Young people who grow up believing in themselves and in their own capabilities will, in general, show constant improvement in their studies, take very good care of themselves with no fear, and also perform exceptionally in sports and even in socializing with other people. Young people who are very certain about themselves are able to make choices that are beneficial to them and not succumb to peer pressure.

Overall, wellbeing occurs at both a physical and emotional level. They are also interrelated; one ends up feeding on the other. Physical wellbeing, especially when you haven't been in the best shape, helps fuel wellness at a mental and emotional level. By the same token, when your emotional health is at a high point, you are able to translate that into physical wellbeing.

The most important thing is that when you feel good about yourself, your self-esteem will begin to climb and climb. This isn't just about looking good, but also having high levels of energy and lacking any serious ailments. So, paying attention to your emotional and physical wellbeing is definitely essential to achieving your goal of being the best that you can possibly be.

7. Changes Happen — and YOU Can Change, Too

Constructive self-respect differs from individual to individual, yet research demonstrates that this mental asset rises and falls in methodical manners over the span of a lifetime.

Researchers, as of late, sifted through various investigations of confidence to outline the normal changes that happen from youth to adulthood. It helped them to better understand how confidence creates and develops our experience of connections, of the important of well-being, of our ability to follow instructions, and our ability to achieve whatever we set out to achieve.

The researchers examined 331 investigations that evaluated confidence, which included 164,000 individual participants falling somewhere between the range of 4 and 94 years of age. Confidence is measured with polls in which respondents' state to what degree they concur with certain statements, such as, "I am an individual of worth, at any rate on an equivalent premise with others" or "I wish I had more regard for myself."

The researchers found that confidence would, in general, ascend from ages 4 - 11, stay stale from 11 - 15, increase extraordinarily from 15 - 30, and unpretentiously improve until cresting at 60. It remained consistent from 60 - 70 years, declined somewhat in individuals ages 70 – 90, and dropped significantly between ages 90 - 94. (Fewer research studies tended to the most youthful and elderly age groups—only a few participants were in the 4 - 6 territory and 90 to 94 territory—so the findings hold less weight for individuals who fall in these age ranges). The outcomes were distributed in the journal known as the Psychological Bulletin.

Each individual has an extraordinarily unique arrangement of life experiences; the patterns we have studied just outline the normal changes that happen. All things considered, the general development in confidence between ages 4 and 60 speaks to significant change. "The combined increase in confidence going from youth to youthful adulthood to midlife was a lot bigger than I expected," says Richard Robins, a brain science educator at the University of California.

The discoveries challenge presumptions researchers recently held about particular age groups. Past proof proposed that youngsters experience a decline in confidence somewhere in the range of 7 and 9 years of age. It was felt that children at first build up an inflated sense of self, which they eventually realize is unrealistic and inaccurate as they set foot on the path to accepting their genuine and imperfect self. This realization, which often occurs to children between the ages of 7 and 9, leads to a significant blow to a child's self-confidence. Be that as it may, self-esteem ultimately ended up increasing somewhat during this time window, perhaps because they become more forgiving and accepting of their own mistakes and shortcomings.

Another past supposition was that young people experience a sharp drop in confidence that can be organized into different categories—for example, testing scholastic conditions, social examination, and the physiological changes experienced during pubescence. Nevertheless, the survey exhibits that all things considered, confidence is held consistently. This finding doesn't really suggest that everybody goes on with their lives experiencing a healthy level of confidence, Robins notes. Changes that occur during one's youth or adulthood likely lead to some issues that make having a healthy level of confidence difficult.

But let's think about you.

As I already said in the Introduction, once you have adopted the strategies we have developed in this book, you will be able to translate them into a winning formula that can hold up over time. The best part about this is that you don't need any superpowers to get these changes.

You already have everything you need to become the successful person you've always wanted to be. Perhaps the most important thing you can keep in mind is: you must act! You can't expect to see any change without first deciding to act.

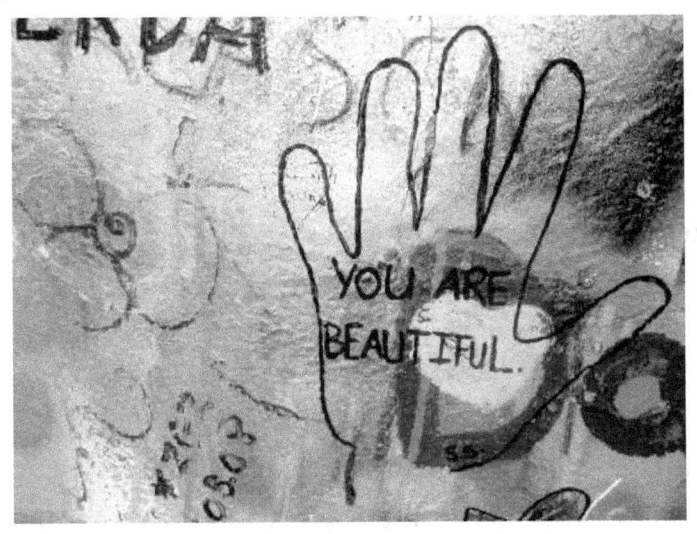

Part 2: Boosting Your Self-Confidence in Steps

Low self-confidence is something that stems from within oneself. The more terrible you feel about what your identity is and what you do, the less motivation you will have to take the necessary steps to construct your self-confidence. From that point, it is easy to fall into a cycle of negative and irrational reasoning, keeping you buried in harmful and inaccurate ideas about yourself. How can you stop this endless loop and start moving in a progressive, positive way? It's a process, and it won't occur without any preparation, but there are things that you can to change and keep it moving.

All of us have confidence. Confidence is comprised of the musings we have about ourselves and assumes a significant role in nearly everything that we do. Having sound confidence is extremely significant as it ultimately leads to you making constructive decisions in your daily life, and gives you the mental strength to be yourself and to have positive connections. All of these benefits would help you manage troublesome circumstances. It's critical to accept the fact that you can change and that, in general, all humans are capable of change. Change does not happen overnight, but it happens consistently throughout our lives.

Though it does not seem doable, if you have a low level of self-confidence, there are various things you can do to raise it to a higher level. It is not inherited, and an individual is not required to depend on anyone but themselves to build up their level of self-confidence. Also, the moment you realize that no situation is permanent and that you will not be able to control everything, then you can start working on your confidence. At that particular moment, you could start working on yourself and accepting that you deserve respect in spite of what others say about you.

You can do this by assuming responsibility for your life, and assuming responsibility for your self-assurance. By involving yourself in physical activities that will improve your fitness, and changing the way you view yourself, you can easily build your self-confidence without external assistance.

There are basic mediations planned for helping you increase your confidence:

8. Challenge Bad Thoughts About Yourself

In order to challenge bad thoughts about yourself, you need to come up with positive thoughts about yourself. This can be done by taking note of at least three things that you are good at. Try and remind yourself of and focus on what you are particularly good at when you are feeling low as they could help you feel better about yourself in those moments.

Whenever you have a negative thought, stop and assess whether it is accurate. Search for evidence. Try to imagine what reaction you would have if a friend spoke about themselves in that manner. You would definitely give them a more positive reply. Therefore, use the same method to challenge the negative thoughts that you get. Think of a more positive thought to replace a negative one.

You need to find methods to get to know more about the way in which you think of yourself. For example, when you are out there jogging or exercising, and your brain speaks to you, saying that it is hard, so you consider going back home and resting—this is the perfect example of a situation in which you can start overcoming your negative thoughts and think in a more positive manner. Thinking more positively enables you to live more positively. It might help to think of a negative thought as some type of obstacle that you need to get rid of.

When we have a low level of self-confidence, we often fear failure so much that we do not even attempt to do something that could potentially result in failure. In order to overcome this fear, think about the occasions you were frightened of accomplishing something, yet you attempted it anyway and ended up succeeding. It could be the first occasion when you plunged into a swimming pool, the first time you asked somebody out on a date, or the time you played an instrument before an audience at school.

This may appear to be unrelated, but think about these occurrences for a moment. We, as a whole, can defeat our negative thoughts. All the time, our brains overstate conceivable negative results and replay them again and again in our minds. A lot of our apprehensions are ridiculous. As Mark Twain stated, "I have gone through a large portion of my time on earth stressing over things that never occurred."

The normal individual has a huge number of considerations every day, and a considerable amount of these considerations is negative. We are continually conversing with ourselves in our minds, so it just generally a good idea to focus on the tone of our internal exchanges. We state and think things, for example, "I am a disappointment,""I can't be believed,""She can't

be believed,""Life is uncalled for,""I am
excessively short,""I can't do this," and so on.
With consistent mindfulness, you can identify
when you are having negative thoughts and work
to replace them with positive ones.

9. Get to Know Yourself/Become
Your Own Best Friend

A best friend is somebody you can trust with
your most profound mysteries, somebody to
depend on in times of emergency, and somebody
to celebrate important life occasions with. Be
that as it may, building up the courage to be your
very own closest companion implies that you can
depend on your judgment and be your very own
source of solace when you need encouragement
or support. Being your own best friend can
likewise be an incredible method to work
through sentiments of dejection, frailty, and
confusion in your life. By developing a positive
self, you can figure out how to confide in yourself

consistently and refer to yourself in times of distress.

Invest your energy in becoming acquainted with yourself. Consider what drives you, your preferences, and your strengths and shortcomings. We will, in general, search externally to make sense of our own preferences, thoughts, objectives, and interests, from social chit-chats around the water cooler at work to Facebook posts and Instagram posts.

However, the more you understand yourself on a genuine level, the simpler it will be to accept yourself for who you truly are as opposed to who you think you are as a result of other individuals, patterns, and conditions throughout your life. Think about how you communicate with the individuals in your life, from your coworkers to your friends and family. Your attitude towards others reflects how you feel about yourself.

When a battalion is going to war, the commander has to figure out long before the day of battle how to defeat the enemy. It is unwise to do so without getting to know the enemy well enough. In this regard, anytime you are attempting to beat the negativity in your mind, it is good to know that self-assurance is in yourself. Get to know yourself well by tuning into the things that are in your mind.

Write down the negative thoughts running through your head and consider why such thoughts would come to you. Afterward, take note of the things that benefit you, the things that make you progress in life positively, and the things that make you happy. On the other hand, take note of the things that restrict you and hinder you from developing positively and note whether they are reasonable or could be done away with. By doing this, your self-assurance will grow in the end.

Fear is a feeling that every human being gets once in a while. It is a component that is necessary for keeping us safe and alive. However, when taken too far, it can start becoming demoralizing and debilitating. Fear causes a lack or loss in confidence in our abilities. When we acknowledge fear, we are able to manage it so as it won't affect our ability to make decisions as well as risk-taking that is vital in self-growth and helps us get out of our comfort zone.

Fear is a part of life; it is completely normal that we experience it once in a while throughout our lifetime. Individuals are not advised to be ashamed of having fear as it is not a weakness. It is important to understand that fear exists anytime that we want to venture into things that are meaningful, but that should not stop us from engaging in these things. That is the meaning of courage. We need to be the drivers when fear comes along as a passenger.

10. Accept Yourself

First: Self-acknowledgment is vital to feeling certain about yourself and your abilities. At the point when individuals give you congratulations, just express profound gratitude as opposed to dismissing them or saying something negative.

Second: Nobody is perfect. Acknowledge your 'blemishes' or flaws and figure out how to cherish them. They are what make you one of a kind—work it! Think about other individuals, too. They have flaws. They are always battling with their character, their life stays a steady process of acclimating to everyone's criticism. They try and please everyone and never end up satisfied with themselves. As people, we will, in general, get judgmental when we like the great pieces of our self and disdain the other pessimistic pieces of our mind. Refusal of the presence of our duality prompts concealment of the negative parts or not all the appreciated pieces of our being; we over and again would prefer not to feel and recognize its essence. In any case, they keep on existing within us— turning a blind eye doesn't change the truth.

This inability to acknowledge yourself as a good person, someone who is capable of anything they put their mind to, results in uneasiness and negativity. Naturally, accepting yourself for who you are and what you have and can accomplish is the start of a bigger adventure; it opens you up to also acknowledging others for who they truly are and what they have and can accomplish. It enables you to identify with others wholeheartedly.

By this point, you should be able to recognize that you don't have to change who you are to accept who you are, even if you are not where you want to be in life. You should also be able to acknowledge the fact that every individual you interact with should also be accepted for who they are without anyone trying to change them. Once you have truly accepted yourself for who you are, you can use your newfound integrity to determine what jobs or career to attain. Both now and in the future. You may have more to work on within yourself and in your life, but this will only enable you to take advantage of your known and obscure qualities. You will have the option to feel another surge of motivation and a strong desire to take on greater difficulties throughout everyday life.

The vast majority of us are unbelievably hard on ourselves. We will, in general, ruminate on our mistakes and disappointments more than our triumphs. Of course, we *have* missed the mark and goofed as everybody has at a certain point. Be that as it may, we likewise have figured out how to beat troublesome circumstances effectively and achieve things that we can be proud of. This tendency to focus on our shortcomings and negate our achievements is a huge contributor to the struggle if accepting ourselves.

List a rundown of the considerable number of things you have accomplished in your life, both small things and big things. You will be amazed at all of the things you have achieved when you look at that list, and you will be shocked to discover all that you disregard and don't give yourself credit for. Keep this list and continue to add small and big accomplishments to it as you recall them or as you accomplish them. Keep it somewhere safe, and read it regularly.

11. Be Kind to Yourself

To have solid confidence in ourselves, it's essential to take care of yourself holistically. A significant number of us disregard our self-care. It is so easy to be kind towards and care for others, but it can be quite difficult to remember to do the same for ourselves. This doesn't need to be a daunting endeavor. You can be pleasant to yourself in little ways each and every day. How you care for yourself directly impacts how you feel about yourself. When it comes to progress, nothing is more significant and persuasive than self-assurance and faith in oneself. Actually, if we need to be effective, self-conviction is a higher priority than insight, ability, foundation, or pretty much whatever else.

Likewise, individuals who have the self-assurance and confidence in themselves are more advantageous, more joyful, have better connections, and are increasingly persuaded and resilient. Seek positivity from others, and ask the people who are closest to you to inform of your positive qualities, gifts, and abilities.

Since we will, in general, be very disparaging of ourselves, getting positive input from other people who are better ready to see your true self could help us. You might be astounded by what you hear, and you may discover that you have more going for you than you realized. Encouraging feedback from others can be meaningful and motivating. The more routinely you do this, the greater an effect it has on your self-assurance and conviction.

Expressing kind and authentic words can feel odd in light of the fact that you only do it once in a while. If you can be caring and delicate to other people, you can treat yourself that way, as well. It just takes practice. Notice the little stuff. Did you send the email that you have been putting off? Did you set aside an effort to tidy up the kitchen or accomplish one thing that has been causing you nervousness? Give yourself credit. Host a movie get-together for yourself or something of that nature to celebrate your achievement. Be benevolent to your brain and work on accomplishing things that make you feel positive.

Tune into your body. Your body is your most noteworthy instructor. If you listen to what it says, you are bound to be more thoughtful of how you care for yourself. Wanting a slice of pizza but eating an apple is healthy, but does not always mean that you are listening to your body. Even though your choice is better for your health in the long run, it is okay to occasionally eat that slice of pizza. It means you are listening to your body and giving it what it wants. In the event that you need to sleep because your eyes can't even stay open, that, as well, is indicating benevolence to yourself.

Each time I get a constructive message from someone like my boss, I make sure to remember that it is not negative in nature, but rather is meant to encourage me to do better and thus feel better about myself. Do support yourself. Give yourself kudos for the things you have done.

We regularly move so quickly during our lives that we don't give ourselves credit, which makes us troubled and frequently prompts negative self-talk. Do kind things for your psyche. Take five minutes toward the beginning of the day or night to relax, listen to music, or accomplish something that satisfies you. Simply make sure to be mindful of your needs and be kind to yourself.

12. Don't Take Yourself, or Life, Too Seriously

At the point when we pay attention to ourselves less, we're ready to see the amusingness in the circumstances, locate the silver coating when things don't go the manner in which we need them to, and explore through the good and bad times of life somewhat simpler.

Defy the dread of being criticized. End the seemingly endless loop—dread causes more dread. Face it and get over it. As Seth Godin stated, "Hit the dance floor with dread. As you move, you understand that dread is, truth be told, a compass—it's giving you a clue that you are onto something." Use that dread as energy to jump forward. Fail deliberately. I don't mean this allegorically. Simply let something become lost despite a general sense of vigilance. This won't just enable you to understand that one slip-up won't murder you—yet it will likewise enable you to recover control. If somebody gripes, essentially smile and disclose to them, you did it deliberately. Intentionally being careless does set you up for surprising mix-ups.

Change the tone, change the discussion. The ideal approach to conquer weight from naggers is by not paying attention to them as well. Sticklers will, in general, think in right-or-wrong terms— either you succeed or come up short. Use silliness to incapacitate their methodology; demonstrate to them life's shades of grey. Figure out how to recognize the voice of shame when it's calling your name. Face that feeling.

Brené Brown proposes conversing with your shame: "This is baffling, possibly destroying. However, achievement and acknowledgment and validation are not values that drive me. My worth is mental fortitude. You can proceed onward, shame. Let go of your notoriety. Your picture isn't you. It's just what individuals see. Try not to give your self-esteem a chance to rely upon your group of spectators' commendation. At the point when your self-esteem isn't hanging in the balance, it's simpler to go out on a limb and be gutsy."

You quit considering, whether you realize how to move or not. You simply start influencing. There are unmistakably times throughout everyday life and certain conditions that are truly genuine. In any case, most of the time, we include pointless pressure, weight, and pessimism to circumstances with our mentality of "reality." One of the best things we can do is giggle - at ourselves, at the circumstance, or when all is said and done.

At the point when we need self-assurance, we are most likely only focusing on our shortcomings and not recognizing and giving ourselves credit for our accomplishments. We get plagued and overpowered by issues and forget that we should be attempting to think of solutions. At whatever point you are incapacitated by your dread of taking on something challenging, attempt to think of approaches to beat potential obstacles as opposed to focusing on all that can turn out badly.

A great many people are much quicker to name their disappointments than their victories. Similarly, we additionally will, in general, spotlight on our shortcomings as opposed to our qualities. We frequently need to depend on the individuals nearest to us to call attention to our positive qualities since we are oblivious to them. Make a rundown of your qualities (to ask your loved ones in the event that you need to) and glue it where you can review them consistently. I promise you that you have much a larger number of positive qualities than you recognize. You have worth and ability that you frequently disregard.

13. Acknowledge Where You Need Change

You may not be thinking about changing or recognizing an issue or the need to change. You may feel moderately content with your smoking, gorging, or medication propensity. You might be, to a great extent, ignorant of the results of your decision to remain in your harsh relationship, for instance, and you may not truly be into getting familiar with the ramifications for yourself or your kids. Generally, you might be content with the norm. You "can't," or rather, don't have any desire to change anything as it might feel scary. Propensities are incredible and have a gigantic impact on figuring out what our identity is and the kind of individual we will turn into.

I took this in, numerous years beforehand, and, from that point onward, have made various propensity changes. For instance, when I get up toward the beginning of the day, I embraced the propensities for drinking a glass of water, making myself some green tea, thinking of something positive, pondering, and after that, making a beeline for the rec center. I rolled out these improvements gradually, though they have had a total beneficial outcome in my life. Pick one propensity you might want to change or receive and start today.

We all have things we want to change, and we have all attempted to make that change in the past. Perhaps you attempted to quit smoking previously but it fizzled. Perhaps you have attempted to leave your damaging relationship yet have been ineffective. You may have progressed toward becoming certain that "this is just the way things are; I can't change this." Or perhaps, your boss, your best friend, your life partner, or your mom has been "irritating" you to quit doubting yourself, quit smoking, stop drinking, and quit gambling. You see these proposals as a burden and a disturbance.

However, now and again, you understand that your gambling issue is causing contentions among you and your partner, and it has caused an issue or two monetarily throughout the years. For example, perhaps you gambled too much one night and come home to a partner concerned about how much money you spent because you are already racking up debt. Possibly you see the worry in your kids' eyes as you sit at the morning meal table, hacking up a lung while proceeding to go outside and light another cigarette.

In spite of this, the thought that you can change has retreated so far into your mind that it is practically difficult to discover. You may be trying to claim ignorance—a refusal to recognize the excruciating reality, musings, sentiments, or outcomes of your concerning conduct. Our actions have ramifications for us and for those nearest to us. We cannot have freedom of choice without the responsibility of accepting the consequences of our choices.

What you don't know could be harming you, or somebody that you cherish. Here is the thing that you can do about moving out of the pre-contemplation phase. Welcome disappointment as a component of development and growth. It's a typical reaction to beat yourself up you have fizzled. Yet, on the off chance that you can avoid beating yourself up and returning to old ways, you will be able to recognize that disappointment is a chance to realize what went wrong and what not to repeat. There are lessons to be learned; disappointment just means that you are trying. Failing and feeling disappointed is okay. Never trying is not. These lessons we learn from our failures assume a vital role in moving forward with our personal growth and development.

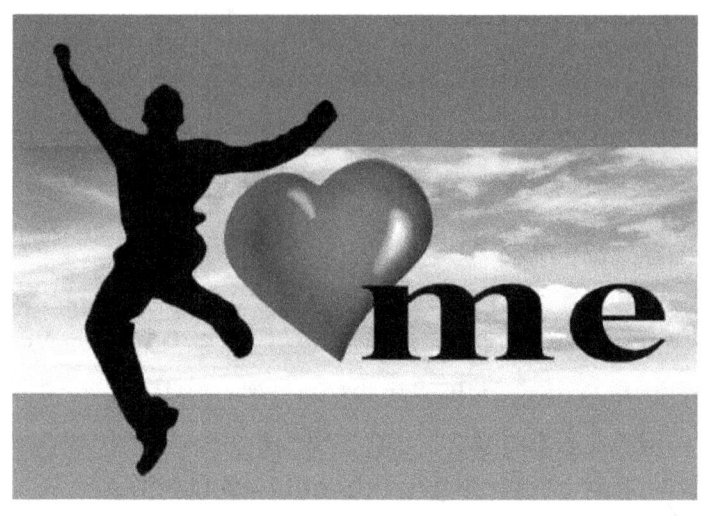

14. Take Care of Yourself

Eating healthily and mindfully and exercising moderately helps the body's regular sedatives called endorphins get released into your body. These endorphins are responsible for the "runner's high" people talk about, or even that rush of proud energy that flows through you as you make a healthy food choice. Overall, the more endorphins we release, the happier we become. Making healthier choices to care for ourselves does not have to involve serious changes overnight. Having a corny dance in your room tomorrow or going for a run around the block today is an extraordinary approach to boost your self-esteem.

By making sure you groom yourself well such as taking a good bath and giving yourself a clean shave can play a part in how you feel about your appearance; this is crucial when you want to grow your self-confidence and change how you view yourself. You are able to turn your state of mind by this totally to your advantage.

After getting a good bath and nice hairdo, it is only right that you compliment it with dressing nicely as this will boost the love you have for yourself, and it will translate positively mentally. This will help you feel courageous and face the world. In today's world, dressing up does mean differently to various individuals. Some will want to wear expensive clothes, while others just wear cheap and easygoing clothes and still look presentable. Watch your sustenance.

Appropriate sustenance is another approach to help self-assurance that is frequently neglected. Our brains are fed by the things we eat. At the point when we eat a well-adjusted diet, our mindsets improve, and we feel much better overall.

An excessive amount of sugar and caffeine can cause emotional episodes and whimsical conduct. Deficient fundamental unsaturated fats like omega-3, for instance, have been connected to sadness. By eating well-balanced diets and food with good nutrients, the body gets the substance it needs, while the mind and our psychological needs get well, too.

Meditation is an incredibly valuable device that can do some amazing things for our self-assurance. Reflection is to mind as exercise is to the body. It prepares our brains and empowers us to watch our musings. This enables us to see both engaging and restricting contemplations. It encourages us to identify the psychological prattle that always goes on in our minds, a great deal of which is negative.

At the point when we reflect, we are better ready to disassociate ourselves from negative musings. Since we realize that the majority of our negative contemplations are not founded in the real world, we can recognize the truth about them and not relate to them. We become aware of our ceaseless personal jabber and ready to watch it calmly from a distance. We find that, in spite of what our negative contemplations and convictions pass on, we are increasingly gifted, talented, capable, and deserving than we suspected. Figuring out how to think transformed me; regardless, I practice it consistently. It is a speculation that will boost your self-assurance and make you more joyful.

At the point when we misuse drugs, liquor, shopping, or whatever else so far as that is concerned, it is frequently on the grounds that we need to escape reality, regardless of whether it is for a brief timeframe. We try to numb our agony and dread. What truly happens is that the impacts of inebriation or being high wear off, and we feel horrible for doing it in any case. We are trying in vain so as to make ourselves feel better when we know very well indeed that it is inconsequential. We feel terrible for having such ruinous propensities and addictions, and that solitary drives us to enjoy our habit much more.

This clarifies why the vast majority who misuse drugs, liquor, shopping, and so on, have low fearlessness, an explanation they wound up dependent in any case. On the off chance that you have a dependence, look for expert assistance, and attempt to destroy the issue. It will do some incredible things for your confidence and certainty.

15. Repeat Positive Affirmations

Positive affirmations do work. An attestation can enable you to replace a negative idea with an increasingly accommodating, positive one and improve your disposition. The manner in which this works is by rehashing, again and again, a positive proclamation that incorporates inside it some sort of conviction or goal. The reasoning goes that if you rehash this frequently enough, you will begin to trust it no doubt, and that changes the manner in which you carry on.

In the event that you present these affirmations consistently, this turns into a type of self-spellbinding as the words will sink into your intuitive and change the way you behave. As to representation and symbolism, positive certifications are short while positive articulations that you rehash to yourself for the duration of the day. They ought to be framed in the current state to be best. Whenever you feel self-doubt infringing, use positive affirmations. Replace your negative thoughts with them. Here are a few examples:

- *I'm competent and able to do this.*

- *I'm cheerful.*

- *I'm content.*

- *I'm shedding pounds, and I am getting fitter.*

- *I'm energized and thankful for this chance.*

Remember that affirmations are best when said with feeling and conviction. It is additionally fundamental that the affirmations are rehearsed consistently. At the point when you are joined with different methods referenced here, attestations can be amazing. I rehearse positive attestations a few times each day, every morning, before I contemplate a decision, and just before I rest around evening time.

Ask the individuals nearest to you to enlighten you concerning your positive characteristics, abilities, and aptitudes. Since we will, in general, be incredibly condemning of ourselves to receive positive criticism from other people who are better ready to see your temperance. You might be astonished by things you hear and may discover that you have more going for you than you once understood. Encouraging feedback from others can be amazing and engaging. The more frequently you do this, the greater an effect it has on your fearlessness and conviction.

At the point when you make little strides and achieve little successes, commend them. In the event that you strolled for 5 minutes today, commend it and give yourself credit. If you effectively composed 2 pages of your novel, praise it. In the event that you ate 100 calories less today than you ordinarily do, commend it. In the event that you ruminated for only 3 minutes today, praise it. Concentrate on what you achieved instead of what you didn't. Keep a triumph diary and write in it consistently. List the little triumphs you encountered and like yourself. You deserve it. This is a ground-breaking propensity that will change your attitude and give you certainty.

16. Relax, Relieve Stress!

Stress assumes an enormous job in confidence. Decrease your worry by investing significant time to accomplish something you find unwinding. This can be anything from taking a shower, tidying up your home, personal reflection through journaling, gaming, working out, and so on. In the event that it works, it works! Smile. In any case, it works. I feel instantly better when I smile, and it encourages me to be kinder to others also. It's a small thing that can have a chain response and not just a useless waste of your time and energy. The way you feel about yourself impacts your happiness level and, furthermore, can make life easier for you altogether.

For example, when you believe in your capacity to deal with what comes, you will be bound to consider difficulties as a test rather than as a danger; then again, in the event that you don't confide in your own capacity to deal with things, you will be bound to consider new challenges to changes to be as undermining and stress-inciting. "Self-viability" is the inclination that you are proficient and clever, and this can contribute both to confidence and stress management. Relaxation brings down the exercises inside the minds' limbic framework; this is the primary focal point of our cerebrum. Moreover, the mind has an intermittent requirement for a progressively articulated action that helps maintain equilibrium. Unwinding is one method for accomplishing this.

Unwinding can truly be of good use once an unwinding process is normally incorporated into your way of life. Pick a strategy that you trust you can consistently do and start improving your self-esteem. One of the advantages of unwinding is that it conquers pressure and strain; subsequently, your physical and emotional well-being will improve. Another advantage of unwinding processes is that they encourage you to be right now and value the straightforward things throughout everyday life.

At the point when you loosen up, you can be cognizant and present; you become serene and appreciative. Start getting a charge out of carrying on with a cheerful life free of pressure. Unwinding is the nonattendance of strain in your body and in your brain. At the point when your muscles are loose and your mind is clear, there is no pressure in your muscles and a sense of relaxation in our minds. Among different advantages of unwinding, that is the best technique to accomplish emotional well-being. It is the best remedy to beat pressure. You can make peace with yourself.

17. Give Yourself a Challenge

At the point when we act and make little strides, we begin to gain speed. We understand that when we start moving, our energy makes it simpler to prop up forward. This is the reason it is so imperative to make a move, regardless of how little it may seem. Just like a rocket dispatch that uses the most fuel, when you start moving, your drive winds up simpler.

Our minds are great at adapting new stuff as they get better when we learn new stuff. Everybody needs an innovative outlet; music, craftsmanship, sewing, games, cooking, website composition – you should simply jump on YouTube and discover a few instructional exercises. All the data you need is out there – it's simply hanging tight for you to tap on it. When you become gifted in something that relates to your abilities and interests, you increase your feeling of competency.

When you find yourself pondering about yourself, stop, and challenge yourself. Try not to give yourself a chance to be constrained by mistaken beliefs. Creative assignments are an incredible method to return the stream to your life. Innovativeness animates the mind, so the more you use it, the more noteworthy the advantages. Haul out your old guitar, compose a story or poem, take a dance class, or join a theatre production. At the point when you include the test of taking a stab at something new, it causes you even more.

Improve your aptitudes through steady learning. In the event that you need to go into business, join up with an independent venture class at your neighborhood school. In the event that you need to compose a novel, read great books, read composing web journals consistently, and take a composition class. In the event that you need to get in shape, at that point, look for guidance from somebody who has done it previously. We ought to consistently be improving our abilities as we learn our new capabilities.

There isn't one individual around who has not failed at something. It is a characteristic piece of life. Even the most successful and wealthy individuals in this world have failed on various occasions. The thing that matters is that they didn't surrender or enable themselves to remain down for a really long time. They tended to their injuries, cleaned them off, and gained from their disappointment. Our disappointments are probably the best life lessons that we will experience.

The main individuals who don't fail are the individuals who don't attempt, and not attempting is a definitive disappointment. Take a look at your past disappointments as important life lessons. Be thankful for them since they have shown you what doesn't work. If you believe that you are bad or not enough to achieve something as a result of your past disappointments, do question this conviction. We all should see disappointment as an important obstacle that improved us. Truth be told, we can actually look at our disappointments as our greatest contributors to our increased self-confidence. Knowing we bounced back from a difficult time helps us feel capable and more prepared to tackle future obstacles.

A significant number of us focus way too far into the future and overlook that a voyage begins with the initial step. At the point when we make little strides and roll out little improvements in our lives, we gradually begin to have confidence in our capacity to make a move. In case you need to shed 40 pounds, you should start small by diminishing your nourishment admission by 100 calories each beginning, middle, and end of a week. In the event that you need to get super fit and exercise 5 days per week, start exercising for 10 minutes 3 times each week. If you need to read 50 books every year, start by reading for 5 minutes every day.

The ultimate goal is to do little activities which you can gradually increase after some time. Once you begin doing this, you will begin to understand that you are able, and you start to embrace your fearlessness. The worst thing you could do for your self-confidence is never attempt it in the first place.

Human instinct is to such an extent that we will, in general, support comfort over uneasiness. We are always attempting to make our lives progressively agreeable while we avoid uneasiness like the plague. In any case, it is essential to recollect that being awkward is regularly proof that we are gaining ground.

It is much the same as practicing and pushing through feeling somewhat awkward as you are in the beginning phases of something new so that we can get increasingly better. We can apply the 'no pain, no gain' phrase here in light of the fact that in any circumstance, we can't improve ourselves and achieve our objectives without encountering some uneasiness. At the point when we grasp distress and remind ourselves that it is for a positive motivation, we grow more trust in our capacity to deal with it. What doesn't kill us truly makes us stronger, and this applies to our self-confidence, as well.

Objective setting is one of the strongest moves we can make in our lives. In addition to the fact that it makes a reasonable vision that we can advance toward, it additionally tells us the best way to arrive. This is finished by separating our objectives into smaller, significant advances. You can use several devices to enable you to set objectives. This is amazingly freeing and engaging in light of the fact that it empowers us to make little strides, which, in the end, lead us to our ideal goal.

Without breaking down our overall goal into smaller objectives, our overall goal often seems much too complex and difficult. By dividing our overall goal into smaller objectives we make a reasonable plan which we can believe in. If you feel like the smaller objectives are still too much for you, simply break those ones down one more time. Simplify them even further. As you accomplish each of your smaller objectives in your day-to-day life, you will gain confidence knowing that you are on your way to your overall goal. Each time you complete a new objective, you are proving to yourself that you can and will reach your overall goal.

18. Take a Different Perspective

Take a look at dubious circumstances from elective points. Attempt to replace considerations like 'Why should I even try?' with 'I won't know unless I try.' By taking a look at a circumstance through an increasingly reasonable focal point, you will understand that you really can do what you need to do – you simply need to apply more energy! Doing this each time there is a negative idea will ultimately result in you defaulting to this sort of energy on the regular. Who doesn't love getting things done?

Our environmental conditions can substantially affect our fearlessness. The individuals we partner with, our schools, our homes, our work environment, the places we visit, all have an influence in building or diminishing our self-confidence. For instance, in the event that you go to the gym, you will be surrounded by other people who are determined to be as fit as possible, and some people that have clearly achieved a very fit status already. The workout machines offer music, fitness coaches, and brilliant lighting to create a climate which promotes the very goal you walked in with. This urges you to be better and urges you to believe that you can do it.

On the off chance that you are attempting to eat healthier, dispose of all the undesirable foods in your home (ones that are not nutritious) and perhaps in your office. Opt to replace those junk foods with nutritious foods. This diminishes enticement and promotes better choices, which, in turn, increases your confidence. The decision is our own; we can choose to engage in habits that make us feel better or considerations that horrify us. How we feed our psyches is similarly as significant as the manner in which we sustain our bodies, and we can choose our considerations a similar way we would look over a menu

In any case, we need to think about our feelings during the time spent choosing our thoughts. Our main goal here isn't to put a fake happy face on everything! Emotions, positive or negative, give us useful information about our needs and wants. In that capacity, they should be recognized, for they are the sign that reveals to us whether we are in alignment with ourselves and our qualities.

The closer we are to acting authentically according to what our identity is, the better we feel. The further away we get, the more terrible we feel. How we respond because of our feelings is represented by our thoughts, and that is the thing that we need to concentrate on today. You are able to pick the manner in which you regard something. Despite what your conditions are, you can start to settle on better decisions. And in everyday life that implies decisions that mirror your qualities and contribute to your dreams. As you practice, you will build up an aptitude that will turn out to be natural to you. At that point, the sky's the limit!

Our thinking is one factor that decides our degree of fearlessness—numerous individuals with low self-esteem do hold limited beliefs that are not founded in the real world. For instance, you may accept that no one likes you when, in reality, there are numerous individuals who adore you and appreciate who you are. On the other hand, you may accept that you are awful at math when, in reality, you didn't make a decent attempt in class or had an educator that was not helpful.

Set aside the effort to think about your limiting beliefs and question their accuracy. Be straightforward with yourself and search for proof that invalidates your inaccurate beliefs. At that point, replace your limiting beliefs with engaging ones that are backed by evidence. Survey these beliefs frequently so you can change them accordingly.

By and by, when I was overweight and insecure numerous years prior, I used to have a restricting belief that I didn't have the self-discipline to be fit, and it sank in my head that my body could not change and my mind won't either, so I will never be fit. When I tested those assumptions, I understood that they were paradoxes. This opened the door for me to create trust in my ability to get fit. That adjustment in my thought framework transformed me. Moving forward, I decided to examine the accuracy of many of my other limiting beliefs and learned to change them as well. This has become a seriously beneficial endeavor in my life.

Each night for 30 days, do the following task:

Pick a peaceful minute and reflect on your day. Record the things you did that made you proud or were meaningful. It does not matter if you only come up with one thing. One thing is just fine. Concentrate on that certain something, and be proud that you accomplished it or feel grateful for it. Notice if you begin you shift into judgment mode and simply laugh at yourself.

Return to the one thing you did that was sure and great. You may find this difficult to do. Statements like, "But tomorrow, I have to accomplish more," are typical yet not accommodating. You are assuming responsibility for your emotions and what matters to you most. You are in control now. You are rehearsing positive affirmations and thinking optimistically, an incredibly helpful approach when building your self-confidence.

The sort of individuals we keep around us influences most of our thoughts, actions, and behaviors. This influences our self-confidence.

Be sure to invest the vast majority of your energy in individuals that are genuine and positive influences, and those that are optimistic about life. Those kinds of individuals can bolster and also empower you through the words they speak and activities they engage in. To summarize an axiom, "Tell me who your friends are, and I'll tell you your future."

Similarly, as we should surround ourselves with constructive individuals who fortify our fearlessness, we ought to keep away from ones that do the opposite. Free yourself of dangerous companions, or if nothing else limit the time you interact with them.

19. Try Out New Stuff

The human mind is great and has the ability to adapt to new things. The more information we expose our minds to, the more we learn, the better we become. Everybody should have a way that they can live out their imaginations—such as music, craftsmanship, move, sports, knitting, trying to prepare new dishes, website architecture—you should simply jump on YouTube and discover a few instructional exercises. All the data you need is out there – it's simply sitting tight for you to tap on it.

All in all, engaging yourself is probably the best methodology for building self-assurance. You can do that from various perspectives, but perhaps, the surest approaches to enable yourself is through direct learning experiences. The Internet is an extraordinary instrument, obviously, but so are the individuals around you, individuals who have mastered or experienced what you are interested in learning, books, magazines, and instructive foundations.

In the event that you need to improve your knowledge quickly, look for someone to guide you and request for their help. A great many people don't set aside the effort to find a tutor and hire them to show them new skills and sharpen existing ones. If possible, find more than one tutor, each having some expertise in the same field that you need to exceed expectations in. Tap into their mastery and get as much guidance from them as could reasonably be expected. A decent tutor won't just instruct—they will likewise *engage* others by pointing out their strengths and boosting their self-esteem.

Identify individuals whom you admire and seek to learn from and get familiar with everything you can about them. In case you need to be a decent swimmer, it makes sense that you would want to examine the life and habits of Michael Phelps. On the off chance that you want to become a successful author of scary or horror books, study the life and habits of Stephen King. When I first began organizing a plan to start this blog, I started reading the online journals of other people who have effectively achieved something very similar. Gaining from those whom we adore and respect inspires trust in our own capacities. All things considered, if they can do it regardless of the considerable number of obstructions they confronted, so can we.

20. Have Reminders That Are Visual of Things That Make You Feel Good

Keeping the things that make you feel good is a way of seeing all the nice things that you have achieved. You could create a section in the house of photos of you and workmates or schoolmates. This could be easy, as we are in an era of portable cameras and memories are easier to capture. Catch all the meaningful moments, so that once you look back at them, you will understand how many awesome things you have done.

There have been numerous studies done on the restraint of perception and symbolism, and it has demonstrated to be a powerful method to help support fearlessness. Similarly how world-class competitors picture themselves winning before entering a competition, one can easily envision circumstances that are positive when feeling fear. Think of a time when you were confident and recall the feelings you got from that time. It's quite important to truly feel it to relive the experience you had and, thus, remind yourself of how good it felt when you accomplished something.

Likewise, you can imagine when you achieved something challenging that you are now grateful for. Once more, feel it with all your being. You can even do this with future occasions. For instance, in the event that you are assigned to give a speech by yourself, shut your eyes and envision venturing to a place that allows you to provide an engaging speech. Picture the speech being one that captures the attention of the entire audience. Feel what it would feel like to have the crowd give you standing ovation; experience the resulting delight.

It is fundamental that you feel as though you were there. Don't simply see it as a film. Be in the film, and consider yourself to be the legend.

Picture the result you need to feel satisfied. Perception works most viably when you feel the truth existing apart from everything else. It likewise works best if you imagine routinely and regularly when you are in a relaxed state.

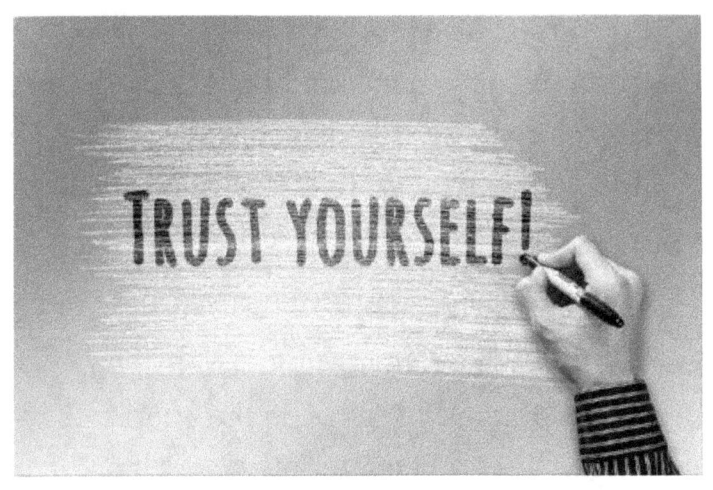

21. Don't Compare Yourself to Others

One of the most exceedingly terrible things we can do to impact our fearlessness is to always compare ourselves to other people. Since all of us are special and extraordinary, comparing ourselves to others just gives us false perceptions of ourselves and creates nonexistent flaws that we begin to believe are real. Rather, we can put much of our focus on the things that contribute to our wellbeing and give us joy. We can quit looking at financial balances, the vehicles we drive, the employments, and the status that we have acquired. Rather, live our lives and be positive about our capacity to seek after the most important goal to us.

Every one of us is one of a kind, and there is no one on the planet that is similar to you. You deserve adoration, so set aside the effort to have moments where you appreciate yourself and feel that affection for yourself consistently. At the point when we adore ourselves, we begin to treat ourselves much better and articulate our issues more kindly.

As we practice appreciation, we are considering all the beneficial things that are present in our lives. As we are all aware, we invest an excessive amount of energy concentrating on what is wrong. Keep an appreciation diary by your bed and record 10 things every night that you are thankful for. This has demonstrated to be an extraordinary habit for some individuals since it compels them to embrace another point of view on life. At the point when you center on quite a few things throughout your life, you begin to have confidence in yourself more.

Approach anyone who is old in age or generally rather insightful for guidance, and something they will likely prescribe is to overlook the comments of other people. I was offered this guidance a couple of years back and applying it to my life has been liberating. An increasing number of people have the tendency to invest a lot of time and energy into trying to please and satisfy others, which is often propelled by the stress of worrying about what others think of them.

On the off chance that we care a lot about the assessments of others, it seems as though we are offering them access to our happiness. The only way to get the powers back to you is to stop regarding what others say about you as truths. This doesn't imply that you become insensitive toward their sentiments and carry on discourteously. It just implies you need to concentrate on your thoughts and feelings about yourself as opposed to the assessments of others. Your joy and certainty in your capabilities ought not to be directed by others. When you finally choose to take this step, you will feel a massive weight lifted off of your shoulders and your self-esteem will begin to improve.

22. Change Your Mental Diet

An incredible method to acquire confidence is to focus on something that lifts you up and makes you feel good about yourself. Define what dignity or integrity means to you, and guarantee that you're living as per that definition. In the event that your life isn't lined up with your character, it will deplete you and leave you feeling awful about yourself. Our psyches have cunning and successful methods for persuading us regarding something that isn't actually accurate. These mistaken assumptions strengthen negative reasoning.

If you can remember them, you can figure out how to challenge them. Here are four fundamental strands of ideas: **high contrast thinking** (seeing everything as somehow, with no in the middle), **customizing** (accepting you are to be faulted for whatever turns out badly, such as a feeling that somebody didn't smile at you because you did something to upset them), **channel thinking** (seeing just the negative side of a circumstance), and **catastrophizing** (accepting the most noticeably terrible conceivable result is going to happen).

So, when you begin to look at the world in terms of possibilities, it is actually quite interesting to see how you might have been going around in circles when the answers to your questions were right there. That is why changing your mind, literally, can have a profound effect on the way you see the world. For example, if you tend to be overly pessimistic, you might view the world in terms of the "worst-case" scenario, when in fact, the likelihood of such events taking place are slim or even completely absurd.

When we come to the realization that most of the ideas that we fear are only made in our imaginative world and not the real world, the truth about them comes out, and we can easily avoid them. You come to realize that despite all the negative thoughts about ourselves, we have numerous capabilities, are gifted, fit, and deserving. Understanding how to meditate transformed me because I practice it constantly. It is a venture that will support your self-esteem and make you happier. Proper sustenance is another approach to help fearlessness that is frequently ignored. Our cerebrums are fed by what we feed on. At the point we have a well-balanced diet, our moods change for the better, and a good feeling comes along.

As you can see, balancing your life and achieving overall wellness is not solely dependent on a single thing. It takes a number of factors for your overall life to take the shape that you want it to take. For example, proper nutrition is one of the factors that are involved. In addition, you can consider regular exercise as another key ingredient. Moreover, your ability to harness your mental powers for the purpose of achieving your goals makes a huge difference. After all, there are many folks out there who live an incredibly healthy life, only to succumb to mental anguish. By the same token, well rounded individuals may find themselves short-changed by poor nutrition and a lack of exercise.

The majority of us know at least one negative individual that we associate with. They are known as the negative Nancy's, and they always try to discover shortcomings and gripe in almost everything. When we get to a point where we begin to gripe, we fundamentally are focusing on the few things that aren't right as opposed to concentrating on all that is right. Focus on your mentality and quit grumbling about conditions since it just intensifies antagonism and doesn't support your valor. Talking confidently and hopefully changes our attitudes and furnishes us with the reassurance that things will show signs of improvement.

Perhaps the best choice I made over the most recent past was to discontinue being a consumer of all TV contents and any form of media that was negligible and not contributing to my life positively. This was because of constraining the negative impacts that influenced me mentally. At that point, I replaced it with watching pleasant movies, reading books that either exercised my 'learning brain' or my imagination, watching educational or playful TV, and sites that were positive. There has been a very significant impact ever since I decided to avoid negativity from my life that was mentally programming me. The majority of things that I view on TV or online usually consist of important things or things that give me the motivation to be better. On the other hand, in the event that you quit reading through romantic books that are trashy and replace them with more diligent books. You will exclusively be able to lessen some great measure of pessimism, which is a major part of your life; you will likewise learn important abilities and become progressively sure.

23. Do Something Physical

This may appear to be inconsequential, yet it isn't. Research has broadly demonstrated that the way we move our bodies does not just influence how we are seen by others; it likewise influences our thoughts. Sitting and strolling with our bodies erect and with our chest pushed out really affects our states of mind and confidence level. This doesn't imply that if you basically sit upright, you will all of a sudden become the most confident individual on the planet. Regardless, it can help, and you will come to find that overtime, it will be a mindless effort.

Have you at any point had a great feeling after getting a good hairstyle, a good clean shave, or a very warm, long shower? We have all had such an encounter. Legitimate prepping causes us to rest easy thinking of our well-being, thus building the pride we have about ourselves and making us feel more confident.

Doing at least a few difficult or consistently challenging things is perhaps one of the most ideal approaches to creating and embracing fearlessness. It's not that I'm proposing that someone runs some long-distance race sometime soon, but everyone has the ability to focus on at least one challenging thing every day. For instance, on the off chance that you are bashful, you could choose to start a discussion with another person—something that would clearly challenge you. In the event that you need to start improving your eating routine but you find it to be difficult as you constantly crave foods that are unhealthy, challenge yourself to feed on one veggie-filled feast a day.

In case you despise working out, you can always start with a lot of sit-ups, pushups, or pull-ups daily. In case you don't have enough knowledge in certain areas of life, conclude that you will read one section of a book each day at noon. Whatever it is, make the pledge to accomplish something challenging that will extend your limits a bit. So imagine a scenario in which it is troublesome. You have the stuff. At the point when you do this, you will gradually, yet without a doubt, assemble your faith in yourself. It may even wind up infectious!

Overall, exercise is one of the most incredible approaches to boost one's self-confidence. In addition to the fact that regular exercises builds a strong body, it additionally improves one's mood, one's perception of themselves, and one's ability to perform certain tasks they might not have otherwise been able to perform. When you begin to work out, some feel-good hormones get produced by your body, like dopamine and serotonin. You will definitely have a better overall appearance, and your mood will improve. Likewise, it will cause an increase in the feeling of achieving something, which supports you believing in yourself and your abilities. You can do so by lifting a few loads and going for runs while focusing on your feelings. Your entire day improves while exercising regularly, and you will be able to notice a huge contrast when you avoid or skip your exercise routine.

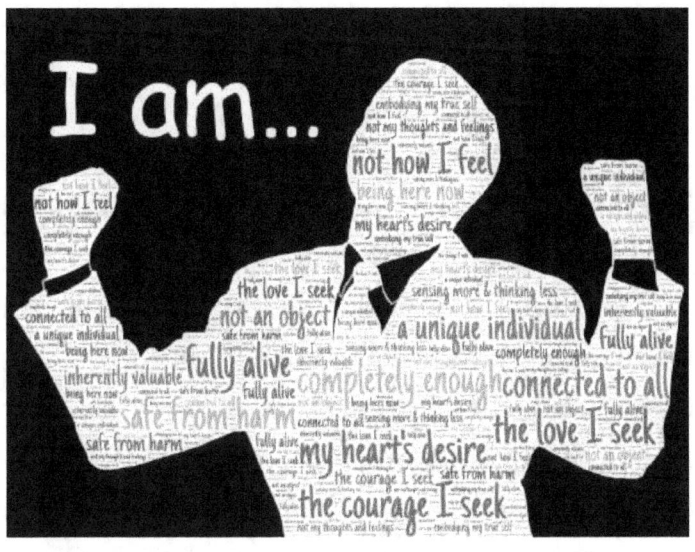

Part 3: Improve Your Relationship with Others

Positive confidence is fundamental to a person's psychological wellness and capacity to relate well to other people. By reinforcing one's self-confidence, one will build satisfaction in their interactions with other people, and they will feel more enthusiastic about their everyday life. However, most of us inevitably have our confidence depend on the way that other people view us.

It is not necessarily the case that solitary individuals endure low confidence, as long as they have, at any rate, one significant adoring relationship in their life—for example, a companion, parent, or kin. "We need, in any event, one significant other who checks our feeling of worth. Our character is the distinction about us that has any kind of effect. It should consistently be grounded in a social setting—in a relationship" (Bradshaw, 1996).

When one acknowledges the significance of confidence to connections vice-versa, it tries building or reinforcing both our very own confidence and that of our loved ones. Coming up next are a couple of proposals for expanding relationship satisfaction and steadiness by building positive confidence. In order to improve one's relationship with others, it is wise to note the following:

- <u>Abstain from censuring, accusing, and
  disgracing</u> – Undesirable connections are
  portrayed by over the top measures of
  analysis and judgment. Persevering
  analysis, judgment, and accusing lead to
  constant sentiments of disgrace. While
  there are a few parts of disgrace that are
  versatile, for example, understanding that
  we are questionable and at times need
  assistance, an excess of disgrace brings
  about low confidence. It causes sentiments
  of "being defective."

It is critical to recognize disgrace from
blame. Both may come about because of
committing an error or having
accomplished something incorrectly. John
Bradshaw summarized the distinction as a
blameworthy inclination signifies, "I
accomplished something incorrectly" while
disgrace emotions signify "There's some
kind of problem with me" (Bradshaw,
1996). While blame attached to particular

conduct may prompt remedial activity, disgrace over and over again brings about sentiments of deficiency, and along these lines low confidence.

It isn't at all abnormal for couples who are contending to fall into a propensity for reprimanding one another. "In the event that you weren't so childish, you'd help more with the housework!"You're so flippant with cash. That is the reason we fight to cover tabs." Even more regrettable, "What's up with you?! Don't you know not to do that?!" These are, for the most part, assaults on the other individual's character and their feeling of self.

They ordinarily bring out sentiments of disgrace or humiliation, potentially working up youth wounds brought about by the reactions of a parent. Regardless of whether you get the outcome that you are looking for from this kind of remark, you could be doing genuine damage to your relationship. John Gottman's examination found that steady analysis is one of the four indications of a disintegrating relationship (Gottman, 1999).

- <u>Acknowledge the other individual as they are; don't attempt to change them</u> - Tolerating the other person's fundamental character incorporates acknowledgment of the qualities that you acknowledge and those that you don't. The essential "huge five" character characteristics are openness to new encounters (versus inclination for the commonplace/safe), morality (versus lack of regard), extroversion (versus introversion), suitability (versus contentiousness), and neuroticism (versus firmness).

These attributes aren't probably going to change much during a lifetime, albeit one can alter their conduct with some exertion.

Reprimanding or making a decision about another person's conduct as it identifies with these attributes is futile and accomplishes more damage than anything else.

For instance, I was once a friend of a couple that had profoundly different habits about tidiness and association in their home. Allison favored a systematic home where everything was in its place, and the surroundings were uncluttered. Joe was the direct inverse; he had a tendency to leave things at any place he last used them and not worry about clean appearances.

A steady complaint was over Joe leaving his shoes in the "center of the kitchen floor," just as papers and a PC on the eating table. Allison was commonly more principled about tidiness than Joe, and this distinction was upsetting for both. She blamed him for being "messy and discourteous," to which he reacted that he felt "controlled by her." This association caused awful fights for both. When the two acknowledged that there is no requirement for judgment on the issue nor was "correct" or "wrong," they had the option to shape social tradeoffs.

- <u>Offer veritable recognition and gratefulness for the qualities that you esteem in one another</u> - Speaking real expressions of thankfulness is one of the six significant ways that we express love for other people. This demonstration additionally has a positive effect on confidence, especially when the recognition is about general traits, instead of explicit achievements. "I love your inventiveness and your creative mind."Your awareness of other's expectations allows me to unwind and not always be known as the upright one." Comments, for example, these have the impact of fortifying our feeling of being entire and esteemed.

- <u>Stay away from compulsiveness in yourself and in others. Acknowledge mistakes as a feature of mankind</u> - At the point when kids are brought up in a culture of hairsplitting, there is steady dread and fear of committing an error. The family principle turns out to be: Always be correct, and be the bigger person. In the event that you were brought up in a perfectionistic family that held these types of beliefs and personal expectations, you may feel that you should consistently focus on the impressions that you give to others. "What will individuals think of me, or of us as a family?"

This unreasonable objective prompts significant misery. It sets you up for an outlandish undertaking since people are flawed. To be really human and real requires the acknowledgment that nobody is perfect. In the wise words of Bradshaw, "Hairsplitting is barbaric." If you don't anticipate compulsiveness in yourself, you won't anticipate it from others. Developed confidence will result in desires for yourself and your friends and family.

In the event that you are involved with somebody of special significance to you, there is an open door for self-awareness. The manners by which you speak with one another can have a positive or negative effect on confidence for both of you. Following these rules can assist you with boosting each other's confidence and, subsequently, your relationship fulfillment.

24. Dogs Can Enhance Self-Esteem

In general, pets can be incredible partners and friends. There are a myriad of pets out there to choose from. The most common domestic pets are cats and dogs. However, there are some more exotic ones out there, too. The fact of the matter is that whatever your choice of pet, you can come to count on a friend who will always be willing to listen to you and won't judge you. Pets are very much willing to accept you and love you with all of your virtues and shortcomings. After all, when was the last time you heard a dog turning someone down? When was the last time you heard a cat passing on a human? What about a goldfish?

Pets are fun-loving, unconditionally supportive, innocent, and delightful. What is there not to love about pets? Past these mindset hoisting commitments, they are sensible. I am not discussing the support they give to the physically or mentally hindered or their support to the profits of breeders, either. They sort of train dogs to provide their owners with the best possible support and behaviors. In reality, dogs have proven time and time again to have a natural inclination to support their owners' enthusiastic wellbeing and improve their life span. They likewise make you feel good and improve your confidence. Confidence is an overall assessment of oneself. Most of us determine how confident we are in ourselves based upon who we are closest to and who has the most influence in our lives. What people close to us say about us and think about us impacts how we talk about and think about ourselves.

Dogs, in particular, make some of the best companions and friends. They are highly intelligent and very sympathetic. Dogs have a keen sense in which they can easily pick up on the emotions of their human companions. If you have ever owned a dog, you know how they can sense when you are down, or perhaps feeling blue after a tough day. In a way, it is a blessing that dogs can't speak. If they did, what do you think they would say? Perhaps they would offer advice and comfort from a perspective much different than that of a human. But sometimes, we don't need advice. We just need comfort.

When a person is feeling trapped by low self-esteem and low self-confidence, dogs can be the ideal friends to get that human out of their rut. Dogs love to have fun, they are always up for play and never back down from tagging along. Dogs are also very protective of their owners. If anything characterizes dogs, it is their loyalty. This is why having a dog can do wonders to the self-esteem of a person. By having someone that they can count on, like a faithful companion, they can build around that foundation. Your dog can provide you with the base you need to build your life around.

Given the fact that low confidence thwarts profitability and self-improvement, finding a viable solution to it is a must. That is where dogs can do wonders for you, or anyone you know who has low self-esteem.

In addition, studies have shown that the emotional benefits that are derived from owning a dog also translate into physical health benefits. For example, dog owners report lower levels of stress and anxiety. Also, dog owners have been known to have lower blood pressure and, more specifically, a significant number of dog owners who have diabetes report that owning a dog eases their symptoms. At the end of the day, there are plenty of reasons why getting a dog is one of the best decisions that you can make.

Here are 4 specific ways a dog can support our confidence.

- **Genuine love** - Some portion of confidence relies upon how appreciated and acknowledged one feels. Individuals with low confidence may need major help and positive affirmations from their companions. This is one part of the social help that a dog can cure. Canines give genuine love to their owners. All owners need to do is be present and take care of their pets, and they will, without a doubt, return the favor with unconditional love.

- **Imperativeness** - Individuals with low confidence will, in general, feel unimportant in their life and in the lives of those close to them. Having a pet that relies upon them for nearly everything directly reverses that feeling. As you begin to realize that you are needed by your pet, you feel more worthy in your day to day life. You feel like you have a purpose. You feel more significant as a human being because you are truly the most important person in your pet's life.

- **Liberality** - Giving adoration, physical consideration, and friendship is a surefire approach to combat anxiety and depression. That delight is an innate part of being a dog owner. A decent owner is liberal with their time, assets, and warmth—all of which make you feel incredible and help improve your self-confidence.

- **Compassion** - Studies show that children and youth who own and care for pets grow to have more empathy than their friends who did not grow up owning and caring for pets. This finding isn't astounding, given that they must be receptive to their creature's needs and generalize this ability to others around them. Practicing empathy toward oneself as well as other people helps to eliminate false negative ideas and beliefs that can cause harm to the self-image.

Owning a dog is a job that involves numerous advantages for enthusiastic wellbeing and confidence. With genuine love and feeling irreplaceable and free, owners figure out how to disguise positive messages about themselves. Those advantages likewise upgrade confidence, with waves of positive change in life all in all.

Overall, owning a dog can be one of the most rewarding experiences in your life. By taking care of someone who needs you and depends on you for just about everything, you can find a valuable purpose in life. The truth is that taking care of someone who is more vulnerable than you is one of the most incredible ways in which you can put your talents to good use. So, taking care of a dog, especially a rescue dog who was perhaps in rough shape before you adopted it, will give you the sense of purpose that you may have been looking for. Moreover, you will know what true friendship and companionship is all about.

So, if you have been thinking about a furry companion, you are all out of excuses. The evidence is abundant, and the research is clear with regard to the benefits of owning a dog. You won't regret having a dog. Your life will be so much better. Even if you are close to your family and friends, you will find that having a pet can foster a relationship on a deeper level that somehow can't be described. In a way, it's a part of the journey toward becoming the best possible version of yourself.

25. Help Someone Out/Give Back

Helping others and giving back to your community can get you out of your typical groups of friends and acquaint you with new individuals. A significant number of these people may progress toward becoming companions, guides, or associates. Other than fostering new connections, being liberal can have a lot of influence that benefits your present connections. At the point when your helping mentality brings about better communications with your life partner, family, and collaborators, everybody ends up benefiting from your newfound mentality.

By becoming involved with and helping different people and organizations, you feel progressively closer with other individuals. People are social creatures by nature, which means we need connections to maintain an ideal mental wellbeing. Interacting with others satisfies a need we as a whole have yet, at times, disregard. Beyond simply the one-on-one associations, the act of helping to address a greater issue or cause (like philanthropy that intends to diminish homelessness, or improve nourishment in kids living in poverty, or give more significant access to education) can make you feel like an important part of the world.

Helping other people confront their own difficulties can put yours into a clearer point of view. This is especially valid if your 'issues' are little by comparison. It's anything but difficult to take things like personal wellbeing, a safe and comfortable home, or a loving family for granted until you invest energy with individuals living in significantly troublesome circumstances. Utilize these chances to develop an appreciation and motivate you to benefit as much as possible from what you have.

After some time, that act of helping other people can assist you with acquiring a new set of skills — particularly if your activities lie outside your comfort zone. Think of activities that are beyond your comfort zone, perhaps something that you have wanted to try but you avoided due to fear of the unknown. Try to live outside of your comfort zone a bit to help others- for example, you could go to a soup kitchen in a 'bad part of town' even if you can't stand food service or do not feel comfortable in that area of town.

At the point when others begin to consider you to be somebody who's liberal and who makes a commitment past their inner comfort zone or circle, more individuals come to you with needs and rely on you to meet them. This is definitely something worth being thankful for. After some time, being viewed as a reliable 'partner' can open new opportunities that you could never have envisioned. Your self-confidence will surely increase.

Researchers have discovered that trust all by itself can be a major indicator of progress. So little successes accomplished through helping other people can expand on one another after some time to create and improve outcomes throughout your life. From a commonsense angle, helping exercises, for the most part, provide you with experiences and skills to put on your resume. This can directly add to your endeavors to get other volunteer or expert jobs. It additionally shows you're a mindful, well-rounded, balanced individual who can contribute to an assortment of situations.

So despite everything you're thinking, whether it means removing some time from your busy calendar to help other people, the appropriate response is an enthusiastic "yes!" It's alright to start small, so don't feel overwhelmed. You can, without much of a stretch, develop your ability to help others after some time as your circumstances, limits, and capacities permit. Be that as it may, by beginning today, you can get a head start on contributing to the greater good of the world, living longer, developing your abilities, and advancing your personal satisfaction.

One other thing to consider is that the most valuable thing you can give someone is your time. Time is the most valuable commodity that we all possess. When you make a point of helping others by giving them your time and attention, you are making a far greater contribution in other people's lives than you think. This is why volunteer work is so coveted. After all, anyone can give money, but not everyone can or are willing to give their talents and abilities for the benefit of others. When you make a point of helping others by sharing your talents and abilities, you are actually contributing to your own self-improvement. This is hardly a selfish attitude; the last thing anyone would call you is selfish by helping yourself through helping others.

26. Surround Yourself with People Who Make You Feel Good

Those you invest the most energy with impact your mindset, how you see the world, and the desires you have of yourself. At the point when you encircle yourself with productive individuals, you're bound to receive engaging convictions and consider life to be going on for you rather than to you. Similarly, as you benefit when you surround yourself with individuals who satisfy you, you can better tolerate when those in your business or groups of friends are negative or extremist.

Do you see yourself as a determined worker, yet your colleagues and group need aspiration? Is it accurate to say that you are looking for that next degree of accomplishment, yet are being kept down by people around you? Distinguishing the individuals throughout your life who are cutting you down is the initial phase in making movements to surround yourself with companions and coworkers that encourage and support you. The ideal approach to figure out who these people are is to consider how you feel after spending time with them. Do you like yourself and prepared to take on new difficulties? Or then again, do you feel irritated, uncertain of yourself, and not responsible for your feelings?

We just have control of ourselves and our own craving for development and change. Some portion of that development and change is choosing the sort of individual we allow in our lives, and the positive effect they can have on us. Helpful and supportive and selfless individuals are real, more so on the grounds that they don't just think about themselves, yet they care about you too. It is essential to them, as much as it is critical to yourself, that you like yourself or that your objectives are met.

Being around this kind of organization will rouse you to avoid descending spirals and ideally convince you to settle on great and sound choices throughout everyday life. Life is tied in with pushing ahead, and it's fundamental to be around the individuals who assist us with navigating towards progress. Having a constructive individual in your life brings comfort. On the off chance that you ever need a source of genuine sympathy, you will realize who to go to. Rather than holding you sad, they will attempt to inspire you, regardless of whether it's simply listening attentively or helping up the state of mind a piece.

Regardless of the amount we need somebody to change, realize they have to modify their own conduct; no one but themselves can settle on the choice to make any modifications in their lives. It harms us to see individuals act naturally self-destructive, yet they should see that what they are doing isn't working and that they have to search for better options. It could be contended that we are damaging ourselves by keeping them in our lives over individuals who lift us up.

We have to realize that we didn't deserve the poor treatment of lethal individuals and that the best thing we can accomplish for ourselves is to proceed onward and truly know in our souls that we deserve better. At the point when we realize we deserve better, we will, in general, draw in better and more advantageous individuals.

You realize who treats you poorly, and you realize who tears you down rather than builds you up. What you may not know is the means by which to expel these harmful individuals from your life. This is another continuous point that surfaces in sessions, and ultimately ends up being a two-section question.

Individuals need to know whether it is worthy of releasing these individuals from their lives. They need some kind of consent, particularly if the individual has been in their lives for quite a while, or sometimes, they can even be a relative. The response to this inquiry is that yes, you can cut off or slowly discontinue content with anybody in your life who treats you inadequately, tears you down, and doesn't have your goals and wellbeing in mind. This is about what is most beneficial for you, and an individual's absence of eagerness to change.

There are immediate methodologies where you explain to the individual straightforwardly why you are expelling them from your life. In any case, they may not be available to hear this, and the clarification might be more for your conclusion than it is for them. This is the easiest approach; however, you need to infer for yourself if this is somebody who you can be so immediate with and that this won't backfire. A letter is another alternative, the same number of us convey what needs be said better by writing a letter and giving it directly to the person rather than attempting to speak our minds verbally in the moment. You can likewise alter your writing multiple times before completing and handing off the letter, and you can spend as much time as you need to be sure you are stating what needs to be stated.

27. Learn to Be Assertive

Decisiveness is simply the capacity to stand up and your privileges, at the same time, also respecting the assessments and rights of others around you. It is subsequently essential inside a sentimental relationship, both to keep up the feeling of your own character, and furthermore, for the relationship to flourish and be solid.

It can likewise be very testing to be decisive with an accomplice. Especially when the relationship is new, you are very prone to need to satisfy the other individual, so it tends to be difficult to stand up for yourself, regardless of whether you feel it is vital. Unfortunately, in any case, behavior patterns learned at the beginning of a relationship are probably going to continue, so you do need to get into healthy habits straight away! Being confident implies that you communicate successfully and go to bat for your perspective, while likewise regarding the rights and opinions of others.

When you become confident, it actually assists you in building your relationships with others, as well as have others put confidence in you. This will come in handy, especially at the point where you are responsible for a big number of duties and jobs in an organization, and you find a number of hindrances. Only a few people are totally confident in themselves. Be that as it may, in case you're not one of them, you can figure out how to be progressively self-assured. Confidence as a whole depends on the amount of trust that you share with any close individual. Confidence gives one the strong will to share and communicate your issues as well as represent others in an efficient manner.

The message being passed across is never the issue; how you choose to pass it will determine how the others will receive and understand it. Having confidence in yourself gives the opportunity to pass the message without fear. If, for instance, you do not take note of the circumstances, the message might actually not be understood.

It is beneficial when one is self-assured as one will communicate effectively. A confident person has a number of advantages. It causes you to shield individuals from walking all over you. It can help you to stop steamrolling others. It can help you:

- Increase fearlessness

- Increase confidence

- Understand and share your sentiments

- Improve your communication

- Improve your leadership qualities

- Make genuine connections

- Add more job satisfaction

Individuals create various styles of correspondence dependent on their background. Your style might be instilled to the point that you're not, in any case, mindful of what it is. Individuals will, in general, adhere to a similar communication style after some time. In any case, on the off chance that you need to change your communication style, you can figure out how to impart in more beneficial and progressively compelling ways.

Here are a few hints to assist you with becoming progressively assertive: take a look at your style. Do you stay quiet, or do you express what you feel? Do you take in some more work in any organization? When under pressure, do you make judgments without thinking of the consequences? Are people comfortable talking and sharing with you?

The use of "I" articulations says what are your feelings at a particular moment without being biased. For example, state, "I do not agree," instead of, "You are wrong." If you have a solicitation, state, "I might want you to help with this," as opposed to, "You have to do this." Keep your solicitations basic and explicit. Be straight to the point. When you come across some issues at any particular time, it is wise not to accept the challenge and give yourself some time off.

Don't stop for a second; give the feedback immediately. If the discussion is restricted by time, keep it simple and to the point. Have in mind what you need to share and tell others. At all times, keep your conversations clear and directly related to the subject. Be audible to ensure clarity of the message that you are passing. Be sure to familiarize yourself with the issue at first. In any case, you can try running the issue through a colleague and friend to hear what their take on the issue is.

Communication might not be fully understood by the use of verbal communication; it is common and important to make use of non-verbal communication to assist you in delivering the message you want to send. Try showing that you understand, even if you do not actually get it. Lean forward in an attempt to show concentration. Keep up an impartial and positive physical appearance. Do not fold arms or legs. You could use a mirror or a friend to practice the show of non-verbal communication and see if you are good at it.

Hold feelings within proper limits. Arguing is hard for the vast majority. Possibly you blow up and become aggressive or become overwhelmed and freeze up, or perhaps you want to cry. These are typical sentiments; they can hinder resolving conflicts. At a particular moment, when you feel enthusiastic going into a circumstance, take some time before reacting. At that point, chip away at resisting the urge to panic. Breathe in and out and try to control your voice.

If you are interested in improving your communication skills, I wrote a book on the subject that you can find on Amazon. Go to the last page of this book and you will find the direct link.

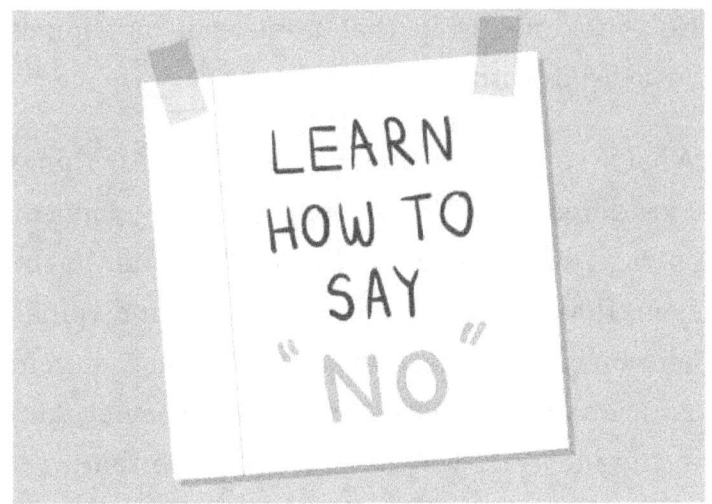

Designed by rawpixel.com / Freepik

28. Start Saying "No"

You can never be successful in the event that you take on an excessive number of responsibilities — you essentially spread yourself excessively far and won't have the option to complete anything wholeheartedly or timely. However, demands for your opportunity are constantly approaching — through telephone, email, IM, or face to face. To remain beneficial, and limit pressure, you need to gain proficiency with the Gentle Art of Saying

No —craftsmanship that numerous individuals have issues with.

What's so difficult about saying no? All things considered, to begin with, it can damage, outrage, or baffle the individual. Second, in the event that you want to work with that individual, later on, you will need to keep on having a decent association with that individual, and saying "no" in the incorrect way can risk that. Be that as it may, it doesn't need to be troublesome or hard on your relationship.

Saying no gets unfavorable criticism. In the event that you decline an offer or a request for help, you're worried that you will sound egotistical or upset someone else. Possibly a colleague needs some help, or a relative does request a favor. You state yes in light of the fact that occasionally, it's simpler to "be pleasant" and keep the peace. You act like all is well, planning to keep away from any conflict. In any case, after some time, being complacent and keeping the peace eventually creates more stress and life issues for you.

Something needs to change; if you don't know where to begin, let me tell you...in some cases, saying no *does* improve the closeness of your connections.

Some of the time, you just need to say, "No." We all have a limited amount of time, energy, and tolerance to give. At the point when you abstain from setting limits, you abstain from being your genuine self and reaching your full potential. This really harms your connections since when you can't be straightforward, connections become less close. It's unrealistic to feel close to somebody when you can't be totally open about what you need. Closeness originates from legitimacy, not imagining.

Additionally, when you give excessively, your needs get set aside for later. You begin to feel unseen, unheard, and forgotten about. You feel like people have forgotten that you have your own needs as well. What's more, when others don't respond, you are left even more baffled than before because you are giving so much and receiving so little in return. Those feelings of disdain putrefy until they transform into is an internal battle. In the case that nothing changes, you might flip a switch and no longer have any desire to even be around the individual who takes so much time and energy from you without ever even offering to return the favor. The relationship begins to fizzle.

Saying "no" to a request isn't childish or impolite when you are trying to prioritize yourself. At the point when self-care turns into a fight, stress does increase. These sentiments ought to never be overlooked on the grounds that they negatively affect your mind and body. Some regular physical indications of stress are headaches and migraines, stomach pains, and digestion-related problems. It's normal and necessary to have and meet your own needs.

Those inclinations are what makes you one of a kind!

One significant hint for changing this unfairness is to think about how you converse with yourself. In the event that your "self-talk" is convincing you that others will be distraught if you said no, you will remain stressed and upset. This sort of reasoning expects the most, and always proves to be false. It's called catastrophizing. Rather, change that "self-talk" into increasingly practical, cheerful messages. Things like, "You can do this," or "It's alright to have needs."

Learning to say "no" actually helps to know your responsibilities, as well as how significant your valuable time is. At that point, when somebody asks you to devote some of your time to another responsibility when your plate is already full, you will realize that you basically can't do it. Furthermore, reveal to them that: "I can't right now; my plate is over-burden, for what it's worth."

Once more, it's imperative to be affable, yet being pleasant by saying yes all the time just damages you. At the point when you make it simple for individuals to get your time (or cash), they will keep on doing it. Regardless of whether you do have some additional time (which, for a large number of us, is uncommon), is this new responsibility the manner in which you need to invest that energy? For myself, I realize that having more duties implies less time with my significant other and kids, who are more critical to me than anything.

It's frequently a lot simpler to pre-empt demands than to state "no" to them after the request has been made. In case you realize that requests are probably going to be made, maybe in a casual meetings, simply state to everybody when you come into the gathering, "Look folks, just to tell you, my week is really busy with some tedious and important tasks, and I won't have the option to take on any new demands."

Rather than giving an answer without even a moment's pause, it's frequently better to tell the individual you will think about their request and get back to them. This will enable you to give it some thought and check your duties and needs. At that point, if you can't take on the favor, essentially let them know: "In the wake of thinking about this, and checking my schedule, I won't have the option to help you with your request as of now." At least you gave it some thought.

In the event that this is an alternative that you'd like to keep open, rather than simply closing the entryway on the individual, it's frequently better to simply say, "This seems like an intriguing chance; however, I simply don't have the opportunity right now. Maybe you could seek me out in [give a period frame]." Next time, when they ask you for help, you may have some extra time on your hands.

The individuals who truly care about you will help you in dealing with yourself. On the off chance that they don't, give close consideration. In the event that another person's needs seem to always dominate and take precedence over yours, that is a significant warning. Solid connections should benefit both individuals, not only one individual. At the point when others keep on ignoring your assertive "no," it might be a great opportunity to bring down your desires or even to rethink the genuineness and healthiness of the relationship.

Saying no doesn't need to hurt your connections. Rehearsing this new conduct will feel awkward from the outset, yet with time, defining sound limits can turn into the new ordinary. Continuously start smaller so you can encounter a few successes along the way. The most astonishing exercise you will find out about saying no is that a great many people will acknowledge it. They WANT you to take care of yourself! Organizing what you need turns into the format for making more healthy connections. Never again will you pull in individuals who can't give back. Saying no allows you to act naturally without a statement of regret, and that is extremely valuable.

29. Stop Being a People Pleaser

These are the kinds of accommodating people whose eagerness to help other people and to do the favors that are asked of them brings about the pleaser being exploited by the individuals they need to please. Companions may search them out when they need assistance with tasks or undertakings that they either can't do individually or would want to have another person do. These accommodating people are driven by a sort of charitableness, and a fair desire to be of importance to other people. With the second sort of accommodating people, be that as it may, their thought process is increasingly self-coordinated.

This sort of pleaser can be grinding to others in their diligent need to "help out" in any event even when their assistance isn't required. They do what they can to help others as an approach to procure approval and shore up insecure confidence. This individual is looking for validation through being overly caring of others. They need to be loved by others and may not understand that the very practices they are displaying are the sort that can actually frustrate and smother others and leave the pleaser feeling burnt out.

In the event that you believe you're an over-the-top accommodating person, or in the event that you have been blamed for being an accommodating person by others, you may benefit by making sense of your own motivation for doing what others ask of you, regardless of whether it's beyond what they may accomplish for you. Is it accurate to say that you are attempting to charm yourself with others, or would you simply like to be of help? Those are two completely different motivators that spring from totally different needs and past experiences.

In case you feel you're continually being relied upon to "be there" for other people and individuals appear to exploit your thoughtfulness, the most significant word in your vocabulary needs to become, "No." While it's a good thing to help others as much as possible, nobody should feel that they are at the "beck and call" of others when they need somebody to help them out.

Advise yourself that sound connections include unity—in case you're generally the person who "tries to get along," yet never gets the chance to settle on choices in a relationship, that is an uneven relationship. Also, when a relationship's example has been carved into place, it very well may be hard to update it not far off. On the off chance that you feel you're getting the short finish of the relationship, support yourself. Be prepared to share a couple of instances of the occasions when you feel you have been scammed. Likewise, be prepared to offer thoughts of how you'd like things to go moving forward. Try not to grumble in the event that you can't propose an answer to the issue.

Understand and accept that your time is just as important as another's and be as loving and caring to yourself and your very own needs as you are to those of others. Assess how you invest your energy. In the event that you see that you are not getting the things you need or it feels like you are continually putting your needs and wants second to others because of focusing too much on satisfying others, make clear boundaries for yourself and respect them. Organize your time and ensure that you deal with your own needs before addressing the necessities of others. In the event that you don't keep your very own well of prosperity filled, you will have nothing to offer to other people.

In case you're attempting to satisfy others to earn their validation, reveal to yourself that the one opinion that truly matters is your own. Going through the motions to win the approval and companionship of somebody doesn't bring about a sound relationship. We might be thankful when somebody helps us out, yet that doesn't really imply that we're going to like that individual as a companion. We additionally may not even especially regard that individual, either.

The most straightforward individuals to like are the individuals who make us feel accepted and like we can be ourselves around them. At the point when somebody is continually inquiring as to whether we need help or asking how they can support us, huge numbers of us will, in general, feel somewhat overpowered and awkward. In the event that individuals are reliably dismissing your ideas of help, at that point, perceive that you might make a decent attempt. Venture back and center more around being acknowledged for what your identity is, not exactly what you do.

Not every person that you need to please is fundamentally going to need to be satisfied by you—it's only the truth that not every person we want to like us is continually going to like us. Try not to waste energy or money on someone not worth the exertion. Try not to be hesitant to request what you are being approached to give in a relationship. The most fulfilling and strong connections are those in which unity and respect are present.

This is how you stop being a people pleaser:

- Acknowledge that you have a choice. Accommodating people frequently feel like they need to say yes when somebody asks for their assistance. Keep in mind that you generally have a choice to say no.

- At whatever point somebody approaches you for some help, it's perfectly okay to say that you will have to consider it. This offers you the chance to if you can focus on helping them. (Also significant is to approach the individual for insights concerning the dedication.)

- Ask yourself: "How upsetting is this going to be? Do I have the opportunity to do this? What am I going to surrender? How constrained am I going to feel? Am I going to be angry with this individual who's asking?" Asking yourself these questions is key on the grounds that, all the time after you have said yes or assisted, you're left pondering, "What was I thinking? I neither have the opportunity nor the skill to help."

- In the event that the individual does need an answer immediately, your programmed answer can be no. By saying no, consequently, you leave yourself an alternative to saying yes later in the event that you have understood that you're available.

- Set a time limit. On the off chance that you do consent, inform that individual of how long you are going to be available. In that way, you can avoid misunderstanding.

- Set your needs. Knowing your needs and qualities causes you to put the brakes on satisfying other people. You know when you feel good saying no or saying yes. Ask yourself, "What are the most significant things to me?"

- Say "no" with conviction. "The first no to anybody is consistently the hardest," These are words of wisdom which are hard to adopt but pay off in troves. When you are able to say "no" in a firm but polite manner, you will be taking needless pressure away from yourself. After all, the need to please others can be far harder to deal with than facing people. If anything, others will come to respect you since your word has value, that is, when you commit to something, they will know that you are serious.

- Sometimes, individuals are plainly exploiting you, so it's essential to watch out for control freaks. How would you spot them? In fact, it can be hard to spot such people because they do things in a subtle manner. For example, they might feign helplessness. But deep down, what they are doing is appealing to your softer side. That way, they can take advantage of your good nature. While there is nothing wrong with being a helpful person who is looking to offer support in time of need. But the fact of the matter is that you also need to avoid having unscrupulous people take advantage of your good nature. This is hardly a selfish act; it is an act of self-care.

Utilize an assertive declaration. A few people, at first, believe that being self-assured signifies "venturing all over individuals," Rather, "self-assuredness is mostly about the association." What this means is that you are looking to foster positive relationships with those around you. At the end of the day, your ability to build healthy relationships will end rubbing off on every aspect of your life.

Try not to give a reiteration of reasons. It's enticing to need to safeguard your choice to disapprove of somebody so that they understand your reasoning. However, this really fires back at you.

30. Get Involved in Team Sports

Team sports are competitive, just like any other type of sport. Anyway, when you engage in team sports, be it basketball, baseball, soccer, or any other type of sport, you will find that being around a tight group of teammates will help foster your self-confidence. The main reason for this is due to the fact that you build and maintain strong relationships, you will be able to build on your self-confidence.

The biggest difference between team sports and individual sports is that individual sports will put you on the spot. When that happens, you might feel self-conscious about your performance. For instance, if you are a runner, you might be self-conscious about not having the best time. Moreover, there is a lot more room for you to compare yourself to others. When you fall into the trap of comparing yourself with others, you will find that it can be incredibly detrimental to your confidence.

Sure, there is plenty of comparison in team sports. If you are not the best player on the team, you might feel self-conscious. But that's where the main difference lies: if there are other players on team that are better than you, it means you have the opportunity to learn from them and improve upon your own performance.

Over time, engaging in team sports builds camaraderie. This sense of belonging builds character and confidence. The reason? Well, if feel like your spot on the team is safe, you know that you can take the time you need to build on your skills.

This sense of belonging is exactly the same as what happens in the military. Soldiers build incredibly camaraderie because they are faced with difficult and stressful situations in which they need to be there for each other. In the military, a team effort is needed all the time. Otherwise, the lives of fellow soldiers can be put in danger.

Of course, team sports aren't a life or death situation. Yet, the same do or die mentality permeates the attitude that teammates need to have. When you build such a close-knit relationship with a teammate, or perhaps the entire team, you can find the right spot to build your confidence.

Lastly, when the team is successful, everyone's overall confidence soars. Most championship teams are built on successful individual performances. While individuals aren't always the best players on the team every game, they all have the chance to shine at any given time. And that is what makes being successful at team sports so particularly useful to building self-confidence.

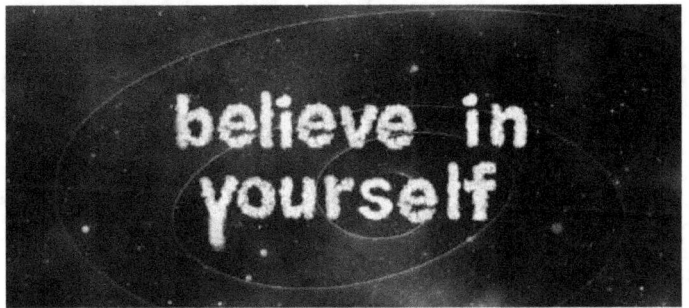

Conclusion

Thank you very much for making it all the way to the end of this book. If you have gotten to this point, it is because you are serious about improving yourself, your self-esteem, and your self-confidence. Now, does that mean that the job is done?

Well, you could take a breather for now. But the fact is that there is work ahead to be done. Having the tools to build your confidence is just the beginning. As you make the conscious choice to put everything you have learned in this book into practice, you will find that making transformational changes in your life are a lot easier than you think. However, don't forget that elbow grease will make the difference between wanting to make a difference and <u>actually</u> making a difference.

The focal point of this work is to examine confidence, its job in human life, as well as its effect on work, relationships, and connections. On the off chance that you have found the kind of work that you deem worthy, I strongly recommend using this workbook to enhance your relations with others.

Also, it doesn't take years and years to do it. Of course, experience is one of the most crucial factors that can help you to become the best possible version of yourself. To me, making changes in your life, your mindset and your attitude takes about 30 days to achieve. But you need to act. You can't just expect to have things happen. Even if you have a great attitude and the willingness to improve, you still need to make a concerted effort to make things happen.

So, what's the next step?

I invite you to sit down and ponder about what you wish your life to be. Picture who you would like to be. If life were perfect, what would you look like? How would you act? What would you do?

These questions are not intended to make you ponder on your shortcomings. Quite the contrary, these questions are about helping you build your targets. After all, if you know what to shoot for, then you will know when you are truly become successful at all of your endeavors. As a matter of fact, most folks are unable to become successful because they don't know what success looks like. Ultimately, you are the only one who can define what success actually looks like.

Please don't fall into the trap of believing that success is measured against what others say, or believe, success to be. Success is different for everyone. That is why you are the only one who can truly define what success is for you. Success might be something as simple as being able to deliver a speech in public, or it might be something as grand as completing your first marathon. But, you will never be able to find out what that is unless you actually sit down and ponder on what success is like for you.

Ultimately, being able to define success means that you are also able to hold yourself accountable. You don't need to put any kind of pressure on yourself. All you need to do is keep your eyes on the prize.

When you achieve what you have always wanted to achieve, you will uncover one of the greatest feelings in life: being successful at what you have set your mind to, solely through your efforts.

If success was so easy, then wouldn't everyone simply be the best?

If success was come without effort then you would see just about everyone achieving their goals with the least amount of effort.

But the fact of the matter is that it takes a dose of hard work and dedication to achieve dreams and aspirations. That is why taking action is the most important thing you can do today, to improve your overall chance of making it. The end of the road is certainly worth the journey. As a matter of fact, the journey is part of the process in building success. When you have achieved your personal definition of success, there won't be anything or anyone what will convince you that you are not the best that you could possibly be.

Final words:

Here we are... ;-)

"Self-Esteem Workbook: A Practical Guide to Help You Overcome Self-Doubt and Insecurity, Gain Better Confidence and Inner Strength — Discover Your Hidden Potential and Change Your Life in 30 Days" is over.

Thank you again for having read this book.

If you are serious about the will to improve your self esteem, I recommend reading this book a few times and starting to put into practice everything you have learned in this book. This way you will change your life!

If you prefer to use the digital version to help you organize an action plan, you can find it on amazon.com.

If you prefer to use the audiobook version, it will be available soon.

I wish you the very best of luck with achievement of your goals!!

Did you enjoy this guide?

If you enjoyed this book, please share your thoughts in a Review. Your feedback is really helpful and I would love to hear from you!

Please leave a quick review on Amazon.com

More books by Dalton McKay:

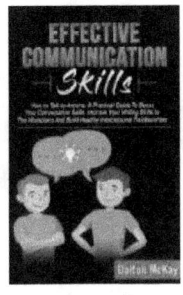
Effective Communication Skills.

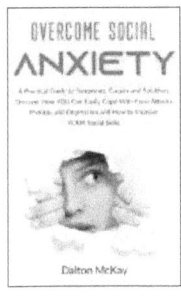
Overcome Social Anxiety.

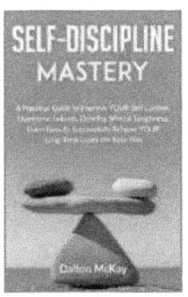
Self-Discipline Mastery.